Day-to-Day Injury Recovery Journal

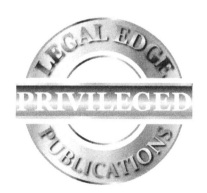

Brought to you by:

Privileged Legal Edge Publications, P.C.

Cinocca Law, P.C. and

Tracy A. Cinocca, J.D./M.B.A.

Day-to-Day Injury Recovery Journal. © Copyright 2024 by Privileged Legal Edge Publications, P.C. All rights reserved. Printed in the United States of America. For information, address Privileged Legal Edge Publications, 10026A South Mingo Road, Suite 238, Tulsa, OK, 74133.

www.CinoccaLaw.com.com

The Privileged Legal Edge Publications Trademark is owned by Cinocca Law, PC. The Privileged Legal Edge Publication books are published and distributed by Cinocca Law, PC.

ISBN 979-8-9899605-2-1 (trade paperback)

1st Edition: March 2024.

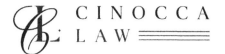

NAME: _____

DATE: _____   **DAYS POST INJURY:** _____

Body Areas Affected & How

Check any & all body parts affected by the accident:

Head and Neck

- ☐ Head
- ☐ Neck
- ☐ Face
- ☐ Ears
- ☐ Eyes
- ☐ Nose
- ☐ Hair
- ☐ Mouth
- ☐ Jaw
- ☐ Teeth
- ☐ Tongue

Upper Body

- ☐ Shoulders
- ☐ Back
- ☐ Upper Back
- ☐ Lower Back
- ☐ Arms
- ☐ Elbows
- ☐ Hands
- ☐ Wrists
- ☐ Fingers
- ☐ Chest
- ☐ Sternum
- ☐ Torso

Lower Body

- ☐ Hips
- ☐ Bottom
- ☐ Legs
- ☐ Thighs
- ☐ Knees
- ☐ Calves
- ☐ Ankles
- ☐ Feet
- ☐ Toes

Sensory Systems

- ☐ Taste
- ☐ Smell
- ☐ Hearing
- ☐ Sight
- ☐ Throat

Other

- ☐ Mental
- ☐ _____
- ☐ _____
- ☐ _____
- ☐ _____
- ☐ _____
- ☐ _____

Describe the pain in your own words: _____

_____

_____

_____

_____

_____

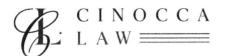

CINOCCA LAW

NAME: _____

DATE: _____ **DAYS POST INJURY:** _____

Body Areas Affected & How

Check any & all body parts affected by the accident:

Head and Neck

- ☐ Head
- ☐ Neck
- ☐ Face
- ☐ Ears
- ☐ Eyes
- ☐ Nose
- ☐ Hair
- ☐ Mouth
- ☐ Jaw
- ☐ Teeth
- ☐ Tongue

Upper Body

- ☐ Shoulders
- ☐ Back
- ☐ Upper Back
- ☐ Lower Back
- ☐ Arms
- ☐ Elbows
- ☐ Hands
- ☐ Wrists
- ☐ Fingers
- ☐ Chest
- ☐ Sternum
- ☐ Torso

Lower Body

- ☐ Hips
- ☐ Bottom
- ☐ Legs
- ☐ Thighs
- ☐ Knees
- ☐ Calves
- ☐ Ankles
- ☐ Feet
- ☐ Toes

Sensory Systems

- ☐ Taste
- ☐ Smell
- ☐ Hearing
- ☐ Sight
- ☐ Throat

Other

- ☐ Mental
- ☐ _____
- ☐ _____
- ☐ _____
- ☐ _____
- ☐ _____
- ☐ _____

Describe the pain in your own words: _____

_____

_____

_____

_____

_____

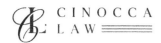

Date: _____   Day: _____

Severity of Pain

Morning: _____

Afternoon: _____

Evening: _____

Middle of Night: _____

Type of Pain   ☐ Throbbing   ☐ Aching   ☐ Stabbing   ☐ _____

Appetite: _____

Sleep: _____

Emotional Well Being

Mood Rating 1-10: _____

Emotional Issues: _____

_____

Nightmares: _____

Fears, Worries, Concerns: _____

_____

Observations

Changes in Symptoms: _____

Side Effects from Medications: _____

Improvements: _____

Deteriorations in Conditions: _____

Medications Taken When & Amount: _____

Limitations on Range of Motion: _____

Impairment of Daily Activities: _____

Help Needed: _____

_____

Help Received: _____

_____

NAME: _____

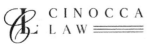

Date: _____ Day: _____

Appointments

Drs.: _____

Clinics: _____

Labs: _____

Therapy: _____

Pharmacy: _____

Visits: _____

Treatments: _____

Date: _____ Name: _____

Specialty: _____ Purpose: _____

Outcome: _____

_____

Conversations: _____

_____

Dr. Instructions: _____

_____

Date: _____ Name: _____

Specialty: _____ Purpose: _____

Outcome: _____

_____

Conversations: _____

_____

Dr. Instructions: _____

_____

Medication Name:	Strength/Dose:	When?
_____	_____	_____
_____	_____	_____
_____	_____	_____

NAME: _____

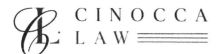

NAME: _____

DATE: _____ **DAYS POST INJURY:** _____

Body Areas Affected & How

Check any & all body parts affected by the accident:

Head and Neck

- ☐ Head
- ☐ Neck
- ☐ Face
- ☐ Ears
- ☐ Eyes
- ☐ Nose
- ☐ Hair
- ☐ Mouth
- ☐ Jaw
- ☐ Teeth
- ☐ Tongue

Upper Body

- ☐ Shoulders
- ☐ Back
- ☐ Upper Back
- ☐ Lower Back
- ☐ Arms
- ☐ Elbows
- ☐ Hands
- ☐ Wrists
- ☐ Fingers
- ☐ Chest
- ☐ Sternum
- ☐ Torso

Lower Body

- ☐ Hips
- ☐ Bottom
- ☐ Legs
- ☐ Thighs
- ☐ Knees
- ☐ Calves
- ☐ Ankles
- ☐ Feet
- ☐ Toes

Sensory Systems

- ☐ Taste
- ☐ Smell
- ☐ Hearing
- ☐ Sight
- ☐ Throat

Other

- ☐ Mental
- ☐ _____
- ☐ _____
- ☐ _____
- ☐ _____
- ☐ _____
- ☐ _____

Describe the pain in your own words: _____

_____

_____

_____

_____

_____

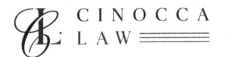

NAME: _____

DATE: _____ **DAYS POST INJURY:** _____

Body Areas Affected & How

Check any & all body parts affected by the accident:

Head and Neck
- ☐ Head
- ☐ Neck
- ☐ Face
- ☐ Ears
- ☐ Eyes
- ☐ Nose
- ☐ Hair
- ☐ Mouth
- ☐ Jaw
- ☐ Teeth
- ☐ Tongue

Upper Body
- ☐ Shoulders
- ☐ Back
- ☐ Upper Back
- ☐ Lower Back
- ☐ Arms
- ☐ Elbows
- ☐ Hands
- ☐ Wrists
- ☐ Fingers
- ☐ Chest
- ☐ Sternum
- ☐ Torso

Lower Body
- ☐ Hips
- ☐ Bottom
- ☐ Legs
- ☐ Thighs
- ☐ Knees
- ☐ Calves
- ☐ Ankles
- ☐ Feet
- ☐ Toes

Sensory Systems
- ☐ Taste
- ☐ Smell
- ☐ Hearing
- ☐ Sight
- ☐ Throat

Other
- ☐ Mental
- ☐ _____
- ☐ _____
- ☐ _____
- ☐ _____
- ☐ _____
- ☐ _____

Describe the pain in your own words: _____

_____

_____

_____

_____

_____

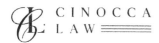

Date: _____   Day: _____

Severity of Pain

Morning: _____

Afternoon: _____

Evening: _____

Middle of Night: _____

Type of Pain   ☐ Throbbing   ☐ Aching   ☐ Stabbing   ☐ _____

Appetite: _____

Sleep: _____

Emotional Well Being

Mood Rating 1-10: _____

Emotional Issues: _____

_____

Nightmares: _____

Fears, Worries, Concerns: _____

_____

Observations

Changes in Symptoms: _____

Side Effects from Medications: _____

Improvements: _____

Deteriorations in Conditions: _____

Medications Taken When & Amount: _____

Limitations on Range of Motion: _____

Impairment of Daily Activities: _____

Help Needed: _____

_____

Help Received: _____

_____

NAME: _____

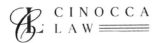

Date: _____   Day: _____

Appointments

Drs.: _____

Clinics: _____

Labs: _____

Therapy: _____

Pharmacy: _____

Visits: _____

Treatments: _____

Date: _____   Name: _____

Specialty: _____   Purpose: _____

Outcome: _____

_____

Conversations: _____

_____

Dr. Instructions: _____

_____

Date: _____   Name: _____

Specialty: _____   Purpose: _____

Outcome: _____

_____

Conversations: _____

_____

Dr. Instructions: _____

_____

Medication Name:	Strength/Dose:	When?
_____	_____	_____
_____	_____	_____
_____	_____	_____

NAME: _____

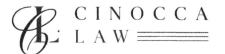

NAME: _____

DATE: _____   **DAYS POST INJURY:** _____

Body Areas Affected & How

Check any & all body parts affected by the accident:

Head and Neck

- ☐ Head
- ☐ Neck
- ☐ Face
- ☐ Ears
- ☐ Eyes
- ☐ Nose
- ☐ Hair
- ☐ Mouth
- ☐ Jaw
- ☐ Teeth
- ☐ Tongue

Upper Body

- ☐ Shoulders
- ☐ Back
- ☐ Upper Back
- ☐ Lower Back
- ☐ Arms
- ☐ Elbows
- ☐ Hands
- ☐ Wrists
- ☐ Fingers
- ☐ Chest
- ☐ Sternum
- ☐ Torso

Lower Body

- ☐ Hips
- ☐ Bottom
- ☐ Legs
- ☐ Thighs
- ☐ Knees
- ☐ Calves
- ☐ Ankles
- ☐ Feet
- ☐ Toes

Sensory Systems

- ☐ Taste
- ☐ Smell
- ☐ Hearing
- ☐ Sight
- ☐ Throat

Other

- ☐ Mental
- ☐ _____
- ☐ _____
- ☐ _____
- ☐ _____
- ☐ _____
- ☐ _____

Describe the pain in your own words: _____

_____

_____

_____

_____

_____

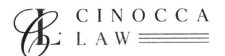

NAME: _____

DATE: _____   **DAYS POST INJURY:** _____

Body Areas Affected & How

Check any & all body parts affected by the accident:

Head and Neck

- ☐ Head
- ☐ Neck
- ☐ Face
- ☐ Ears
- ☐ Eyes
- ☐ Nose
- ☐ Hair
- ☐ Mouth
- ☐ Jaw
- ☐ Teeth
- ☐ Tongue

Upper Body

- ☐ Shoulders
- ☐ Back
- ☐ Upper Back
- ☐ Lower Back
- ☐ Arms
- ☐ Elbows
- ☐ Hands
- ☐ Wrists
- ☐ Fingers
- ☐ Chest
- ☐ Sternum
- ☐ Torso

Lower Body

- ☐ Hips
- ☐ Bottom
- ☐ Legs
- ☐ Thighs
- ☐ Knees
- ☐ Calves
- ☐ Ankles
- ☐ Feet
- ☐ Toes

Sensory Systems

- ☐ Taste
- ☐ Smell
- ☐ Hearing
- ☐ Sight
- ☐ Throat

Other

- ☐ Mental
- ☐ _____
- ☐ _____
- ☐ _____
- ☐ _____
- ☐ _____
- ☐ _____

Describe the pain in your own words: _____

_____

_____

_____

_____

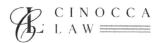

Date: _____   Day: _____

Severity of Pain

Morning: _____

Afternoon: _____

Evening: _____

Middle of Night: _____

Type of Pain   ☐ Throbbing   ☐ Aching   ☐ Stabbing   ☐ _____

Appetite: _____

Sleep: _____

Emotional Well Being

Mood Rating 1-10: _____

Emotional Issues: _____

_____

Nightmares: _____

Fears, Worries, Concerns: _____

_____

Observations

Changes in Symptoms: _____

Side Effects from Medications: _____

Improvements: _____

Deteriorations in Conditions: _____

Medications Taken When & Amount: _____

Limitations on Range of Motion: _____

Impairment of Daily Activities: _____

Help Needed: _____

_____

Help Received: _____

_____

NAME: _____

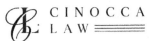

Date: _____ Day: _____

Appointments

Drs.: _____

Clinics: _____

Labs: _____

Therapy: _____

Pharmacy: _____

Visits: _____

Treatments: _____

Date: _____ Name: _____

Specialty: _____ Purpose: _____

Outcome: _____

_____

Conversations: _____

_____

Dr. Instructions: _____

_____

Date: _____ Name: _____

Specialty: _____ Purpose: _____

Outcome: _____

_____

Conversations: _____

_____

Dr. Instructions: _____

_____

Medication Name:	Strength/Dose:	When?
_____	_____	_____
_____	_____	_____
_____	_____	_____

NAME: _____

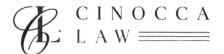

CINOCCA LAW

Personal and Confidential Communication Subject to
Attorney Client and Work Product Privilege

NAME: _____

DATE: _____ **DAYS POST INJURY:** _____

Body Areas Affected & How

Check any & all body parts affected by the accident:

Head and Neck

- ☐ Head
- ☐ Neck
- ☐ Face
- ☐ Ears
- ☐ Eyes
- ☐ Nose
- ☐ Hair
- ☐ Mouth
- ☐ Jaw
- ☐ Teeth
- ☐ Tongue

Upper Body

- ☐ Shoulders
- ☐ Back
- ☐ Upper Back
- ☐ Lower Back
- ☐ Arms
- ☐ Elbows
- ☐ Hands
- ☐ Wrists
- ☐ Fingers
- ☐ Chest
- ☐ Sternum
- ☐ Torso

Lower Body

- ☐ Hips
- ☐ Bottom
- ☐ Legs
- ☐ Thighs
- ☐ Knees
- ☐ Calves
- ☐ Ankles
- ☐ Feet
- ☐ Toes

Sensory Systems

- ☐ Taste
- ☐ Smell
- ☐ Hearing
- ☐ Sight
- ☐ Throat

Other

- ☐ Mental
- ☐ _____
- ☐ _____
- ☐ _____
- ☐ _____
- ☐ _____
- ☐ _____

Describe the pain in your own words: _____

_____

_____

_____

_____

_____

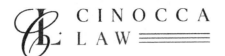

CINOCCA LAW

Personal and Confidential Communication Subject to Attorney Client and Work Product Privilege

NAME: _____

DATE: _____   DAYS POST INJURY: _____

Body Areas Affected & How

Check any & all body parts affected by the accident:

Head and Neck
- ☐ Head
- ☐ Neck
- ☐ Face
- ☐ Ears
- ☐ Eyes
- ☐ Nose
- ☐ Hair
- ☐ Mouth
- ☐ Jaw
- ☐ Teeth
- ☐ Tongue

Upper Body
- ☐ Shoulders
- ☐ Back
- ☐ Upper Back
- ☐ Lower Back
- ☐ Arms
- ☐ Elbows
- ☐ Hands
- ☐ Wrists
- ☐ Fingers
- ☐ Chest
- ☐ Sternum
- ☐ Torso

Lower Body
- ☐ Hips
- ☐ Bottom
- ☐ Legs
- ☐ Thighs
- ☐ Knees
- ☐ Calves
- ☐ Ankles
- ☐ Feet
- ☐ Toes

Sensory Systems
- ☐ Taste
- ☐ Smell
- ☐ Hearing
- ☐ Sight
- ☐ Throat

Other
- ☐ Mental
- ☐ _____
- ☐ _____
- ☐ _____
- ☐ _____
- ☐ _____
- ☐ _____

Describe the pain in your own words: _____

_____

_____

_____

_____

_____

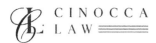

Date: _____ Day: _____

Severity of Pain

Morning: _____

Afternoon: _____

Evening: _____

Middle of Night: _____

Type of Pain ☐ Throbbing ☐ Aching ☐ Stabbing ☐ _____

Appetite: _____

Sleep: _____

Emotional Well Being

Mood Rating 1-10: _____

Emotional Issues: _____

_____

Nightmares: _____

Fears, Worries, Concerns: _____

_____

Observations

Changes in Symptoms: _____

Side Effects from Medications: _____

Improvements: _____

Deteriorations in Conditions: _____

Medications Taken When & Amount: _____

Limitations on Range of Motion: _____

Impairment of Daily Activities: _____

Help Needed: _____

_____

Help Received: _____

_____

NAME: _____

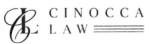

Date: _____   Day: _____

Appointments

Drs.: _____

Clinics: _____

Labs: _____

Therapy: _____

Pharmacy: _____

Visits: _____

Treatments: _____

Date: _____   Name: _____

Specialty: _____   Purpose: _____

Outcome: _____

_____

Conversations: _____

_____

Dr. Instructions: _____

_____

Date: _____   Name: _____

Specialty: _____   Purpose: _____

Outcome: _____

_____

Conversations: _____

_____

Dr. Instructions: _____

_____

Medication Name:	Strength/Dose:	When?
_____	_____	_____
_____	_____	_____
_____	_____	_____

NAME: _____

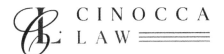

NAME: _____

DATE: _____ **DAYS POST INJURY:** _____

Body Areas Affected & How

Check any & all body parts affected by the accident:

Head and Neck
- ☐ Head
- ☐ Neck
- ☐ Face
- ☐ Ears
- ☐ Eyes
- ☐ Nose
- ☐ Hair
- ☐ Mouth
- ☐ Jaw
- ☐ Teeth
- ☐ Tongue

Upper Body
- ☐ Shoulders
- ☐ Back
- ☐ Upper Back
- ☐ Lower Back
- ☐ Arms
- ☐ Elbows
- ☐ Hands
- ☐ Wrists
- ☐ Fingers
- ☐ Chest
- ☐ Sternum
- ☐ Torso

Lower Body
- ☐ Hips
- ☐ Bottom
- ☐ Legs
- ☐ Thighs
- ☐ Knees
- ☐ Calves
- ☐ Ankles
- ☐ Feet
- ☐ Toes

Sensory Systems
- ☐ Taste
- ☐ Smell
- ☐ Hearing
- ☐ Sight
- ☐ Throat

Other
- ☐ Mental
- ☐ _____
- ☐ _____
- ☐ _____
- ☐ _____
- ☐ _____
- ☐ _____

Describe the pain in your own words: _____

_____

_____

_____

_____

_____

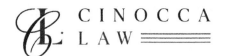

CINOCCA
LAW

Personal and Confidential Communication Subject to Attorney Client and Work Product Privilege

NAME: _____

DATE: _____ **DAYS POST INJURY:** _____

Body Areas Affected & How

Check any & all body parts affected by the accident:

Head and Neck
- ☐ Head
- ☐ Neck
- ☐ Face
- ☐ Ears
- ☐ Eyes
- ☐ Nose
- ☐ Hair
- ☐ Mouth
- ☐ Jaw
- ☐ Teeth
- ☐ Tongue

Upper Body
- ☐ Shoulders
- ☐ Back
- ☐ Upper Back
- ☐ Lower Back
- ☐ Arms
- ☐ Elbows
- ☐ Hands
- ☐ Wrists
- ☐ Fingers
- ☐ Chest
- ☐ Sternum
- ☐ Torso

Lower Body
- ☐ Hips
- ☐ Bottom
- ☐ Legs
- ☐ Thighs
- ☐ Knees
- ☐ Calves
- ☐ Ankles
- ☐ Feet
- ☐ Toes

Sensory Systems
- ☐ Taste
- ☐ Smell
- ☐ Hearing
- ☐ Sight
- ☐ Throat

Other
- ☐ Mental
- ☐ _____
- ☐ _____
- ☐ _____
- ☐ _____
- ☐ _____
- ☐ _____

Describe the pain in your own words: _____

_____

_____

_____

_____

_____

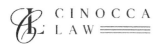

Date: _____   Day: _____

Severity of Pain

Morning: _____

Afternoon: _____

Evening: _____

Middle of Night: _____

Type of Pain   ☐ Throbbing   ☐ Aching   ☐ Stabbing   ☐ _____

Appetite: _____

Sleep: _____

Emotional Well Being

Mood Rating 1-10: _____

Emotional Issues: _____

_____

Nightmares: _____

Fears, Worries, Concerns: _____

_____

Observations

Changes in Symptoms: _____

Side Effects from Medications: _____

Improvements: _____

Deteriorations in Conditions: _____

Medications Taken When & Amount: _____

Limitations on Range of Motion: _____

Impairment of Daily Activities: _____

Help Needed: _____

_____

Help Received: _____

_____

NAME: _____

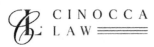

Appointments

Drs.:_____

Clinics: _____

Labs: _____

Therapy: _____

Pharmacy: _____

Visits: _____

Treatments:_____

Date: _____   Name: _____

Specialty: _____   Purpose: _____

Outcome: _____

_____

Conversations: _____

_____

Dr. Instructions: _____

_____

Date: _____   Name: _____

Specialty: _____   Purpose: _____

Outcome: _____

_____

Conversations: _____

_____

Dr. Instructions: _____

_____

Medication Name:	Strength/Dose:	When?
_____	_____	_____
_____	_____	_____
_____	_____	_____

NAME: _____

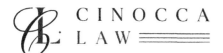

NAME: _____

DATE: _____   **DAYS POST INJURY:** _____

Body Areas Affected & How

Check any & all body parts affected by the accident:

Head and Neck

- ☐ Head
- ☐ Neck
- ☐ Face
- ☐ Ears
- ☐ Eyes
- ☐ Nose
- ☐ Hair
- ☐ Mouth
- ☐ Jaw
- ☐ Teeth
- ☐ Tongue

Upper Body

- ☐ Shoulders
- ☐ Back
- ☐ Upper Back
- ☐ Lower Back
- ☐ Arms
- ☐ Elbows
- ☐ Hands
- ☐ Wrists
- ☐ Fingers
- ☐ Chest
- ☐ Sternum
- ☐ Torso

Lower Body

- ☐ Hips
- ☐ Bottom
- ☐ Legs
- ☐ Thighs
- ☐ Knees
- ☐ Calves
- ☐ Ankles
- ☐ Feet
- ☐ Toes

Sensory Systems

- ☐ Taste
- ☐ Smell
- ☐ Hearing
- ☐ Sight
- ☐ Throat

Other

- ☐ Mental
- ☐ _____
- ☐ _____
- ☐ _____
- ☐ _____
- ☐ _____
- ☐ _____

Describe the pain in your own words: _____

_____

_____

_____

_____

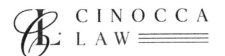

CINOCCA
LAW

NAME: _____

DATE: _____   **DAYS POST INJURY:** _____

Body Areas Affected & How

Check any & all body parts affected by the accident:

Head and Neck

- ☐ Head
- ☐ Neck
- ☐ Face
- ☐ Ears
- ☐ Eyes
- ☐ Nose
- ☐ Hair
- ☐ Mouth
- ☐ Jaw
- ☐ Teeth
- ☐ Tongue

Upper Body

- ☐ Shoulders
- ☐ Back
- ☐ Upper Back
- ☐ Lower Back
- ☐ Arms
- ☐ Elbows
- ☐ Hands
- ☐ Wrists
- ☐ Fingers
- ☐ Chest
- ☐ Sternum
- ☐ Torso

Lower Body

- ☐ Hips
- ☐ Bottom
- ☐ Legs
- ☐ Thighs
- ☐ Knees
- ☐ Calves
- ☐ Ankles
- ☐ Feet
- ☐ Toes

Sensory Systems

- ☐ Taste
- ☐ Smell
- ☐ Hearing
- ☐ Sight
- ☐ Throat

Other

- ☐ Mental
- ☐ _____
- ☐ _____
- ☐ _____
- ☐ _____
- ☐ _____
- ☐ _____

Describe the pain in your own words: _____

_____

_____

_____

_____

_____

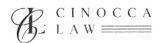

Date: _____ Day: _____

Severity of Pain

Morning: _____

Afternoon: _____

Evening: _____

Middle of Night: _____

Type of Pain ☐ Throbbing ☐ Aching ☐ Stabbing ☐ _____

Appetite: _____

Sleep: _____

Emotional Well Being

Mood Rating 1-10: _____

Emotional Issues: _____

_____

Nightmares: _____

Fears, Worries, Concerns: _____

_____

Observations

Changes in Symptoms: _____

Side Effects from Medications: _____

Improvements: _____

Deteriorations in Conditions: _____

Medications Taken When & Amount: _____

Limitations on Range of Motion: _____

Impairment of Daily Activities: _____

Help Needed: _____

_____

Help Received: _____

_____

NAME: _____

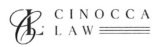

Date: _____   Day: _____

Appointments

Drs.:_____

Clinics: _____

Labs: _____

Therapy: _____

Pharmacy: _____

Visits: _____

Treatments:_____

Date: _____   Name: _____

Specialty: _____   Purpose: _____

Outcome: _____

_____

Conversations: _____

_____

Dr. Instructions: _____

_____

Date: _____   Name: _____

Specialty: _____   Purpose: _____

Outcome: _____

_____

Conversations: _____

_____

Dr. Instructions: _____

_____

Medication Name:	Strength/Dose:	When?
_____	_____	_____
_____	_____	_____
_____	_____	_____

NAME: _____

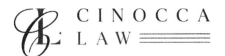

**C I N O C C A
L A W**

*Personal and Confidential Communication Subject to
Attorney Client and Work Product Privilege*

NAME: _____

DATE: _____   **DAYS POST INJURY:** _____

Body Areas Affected & How

Check any & all body parts affected by the accident:

Head and Neck

☐ Head
☐ Neck
☐ Face
☐ Ears
☐ Eyes
☐ Nose
☐ Hair
☐ Mouth
☐ Jaw
☐ Teeth
☐ Tongue

Upper Body

☐ Shoulders
☐ Back
☐ Upper Back
☐ Lower Back
☐ Arms
☐ Elbows
☐ Hands
☐ Wrists
☐ Fingers
☐ Chest
☐ Sternum
☐ Torso

Lower Body

☐ Hips
☐ Bottom
☐ Legs
☐ Thighs
☐ Knees
☐ Calves
☐ Ankles
☐ Feet
☐ Toes

Sensory Systems

☐ Taste
☐ Smell
☐ Hearing
☐ Sight
☐ Throat

Other

☐ Mental
☐ _____
☐ _____
☐ _____
☐ _____
☐ _____
☐ _____

Describe the pain in your own words: _____

_____

_____

_____

_____

_____

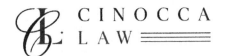

CINOCCA LAW

NAME: _____

DATE: _____ DAYS POST INJURY: _____

Body Areas Affected & How

Check any & all body parts affected by the accident:

Head and Neck

- ☐ Head
- ☐ Neck
- ☐ Face
- ☐ Ears
- ☐ Eyes
- ☐ Nose
- ☐ Hair
- ☐ Mouth
- ☐ Jaw
- ☐ Teeth
- ☐ Tongue

Upper Body

- ☐ Shoulders
- ☐ Back
- ☐ Upper Back
- ☐ Lower Back
- ☐ Arms
- ☐ Elbows
- ☐ Hands
- ☐ Wrists
- ☐ Fingers
- ☐ Chest
- ☐ Sternum
- ☐ Torso

Lower Body

- ☐ Hips
- ☐ Bottom
- ☐ Legs
- ☐ Thighs
- ☐ Knees
- ☐ Calves
- ☐ Ankles
- ☐ Feet
- ☐ Toes

Sensory Systems

- ☐ Taste
- ☐ Smell
- ☐ Hearing
- ☐ Sight
- ☐ Throat

Other

- ☐ Mental
- ☐ _____
- ☐ _____
- ☐ _____
- ☐ _____
- ☐ _____
- ☐ _____

Describe the pain in your own words: _____

_____

_____

_____

_____

_____

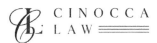

Date: _____ Day: _____

Severity of Pain

Morning: _____

Afternoon: _____

Evening: _____

Middle of Night: _____

Type of Pain   ☐ Throbbing   ☐ Aching   ☐ Stabbing   ☐ _____

Appetite: _____

Sleep: _____

Emotional Well Being

Mood Rating 1-10: _____

Emotional Issues: _____

_____

Nightmares: _____

Fears, Worries, Concerns: _____

_____

Observations

Changes in Symptoms: _____

Side Effects from Medications: _____

Improvements: _____

Deteriorations in Conditions: _____

Medications Taken When & Amount: _____

Limitations on Range of Motion: _____

Impairment of Daily Activities: _____

Help Needed: _____

_____

Help Received: _____

_____

NAME: _____

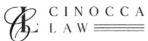

Date: _____   Day: _____

Appointments

Drs.: _____

Clinics: _____

Labs: _____

Therapy: _____

Pharmacy: _____

Visits: _____

Treatments: _____

Date: _____   Name: _____

Specialty: _____   Purpose: _____

Outcome: _____

_____

Conversations: _____

_____

Dr. Instructions: _____

_____

Date: _____   Name: _____

Specialty: _____   Purpose: _____

Outcome: _____

_____

Conversations: _____

_____

Dr. Instructions: _____

_____

Medication Name:	Strength/Dose:	When?
_____	_____	_____
_____	_____	_____
_____	_____	_____

NAME: _____

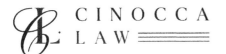

Personal and Confidential Communication Subject to
Attorney Client and Work Product Privilege

NAME: _____

DATE: _____ **DAYS POST INJURY:** _____

Body Areas Affected & How

Check any & all body parts affected by the accident:

Head and Neck

- ☐ Head
- ☐ Neck
- ☐ Face
- ☐ Ears
- ☐ Eyes
- ☐ Nose
- ☐ Hair
- ☐ Mouth
- ☐ Jaw
- ☐ Teeth
- ☐ Tongue

Upper Body

- ☐ Shoulders
- ☐ Back
- ☐ Upper Back
- ☐ Lower Back
- ☐ Arms
- ☐ Elbows
- ☐ Hands
- ☐ Wrists
- ☐ Fingers
- ☐ Chest
- ☐ Sternum
- ☐ Torso

Lower Body

- ☐ Hips
- ☐ Bottom
- ☐ Legs
- ☐ Thighs
- ☐ Knees
- ☐ Calves
- ☐ Ankles
- ☐ Feet
- ☐ Toes

Sensory Systems

- ☐ Taste
- ☐ Smell
- ☐ Hearing
- ☐ Sight
- ☐ Throat

Other

- ☐ Mental
- ☐ _____
- ☐ _____
- ☐ _____
- ☐ _____
- ☐ _____
- ☐ _____

Describe the pain in your own words: _____

_____

_____

_____

_____

_____

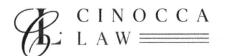

NAME: _____

DATE: _____ **DAYS POST INJURY:** _____

Body Areas Affected & How

Check any & all body parts affected by the accident:

Head and Neck

- ☐ Head
- ☐ Neck
- ☐ Face
- ☐ Ears
- ☐ Eyes
- ☐ Nose
- ☐ Hair
- ☐ Mouth
- ☐ Jaw
- ☐ Teeth
- ☐ Tongue

Upper Body

- ☐ Shoulders
- ☐ Back
- ☐ Upper Back
- ☐ Lower Back
- ☐ Arms
- ☐ Elbows
- ☐ Hands
- ☐ Wrists
- ☐ Fingers
- ☐ Chest
- ☐ Sternum
- ☐ Torso

Lower Body

- ☐ Hips
- ☐ Bottom
- ☐ Legs
- ☐ Thighs
- ☐ Knees
- ☐ Calves
- ☐ Ankles
- ☐ Feet
- ☐ Toes

Sensory Systems

- ☐ Taste
- ☐ Smell
- ☐ Hearing
- ☐ Sight
- ☐ Throat

Other

- ☐ Mental
- ☐ _____
- ☐ _____
- ☐ _____
- ☐ _____
- ☐ _____
- ☐ _____

Describe the pain in your own words: _____

_____

_____

_____

_____

_____

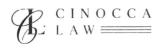

Date: _____ Day: _____

Severity of Pain

Morning: _____

Afternoon: _____

Evening: _____

Middle of Night: _____

Type of Pain   ☐ Throbbing   ☐ Aching   ☐ Stabbing   ☐ _____

Appetite: _____

Sleep: _____

Emotional Well Being

Mood Rating 1-10: _____

Emotional Issues: _____

_____

Nightmares: _____

Fears, Worries, Concerns: _____

_____

Observations

Changes in Symptoms: _____

Side Effects from Medications: _____

Improvements: _____

Deteriorations in Conditions: _____

Medications Taken When & Amount: _____

Limitations on Range of Motion: _____

Impairment of Daily Activities: _____

Help Needed: _____

_____

Help Received: _____

_____

NAME: _____

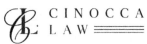

Date: _____ Day: _____

Appointments

Drs.:_____

Clinics: _____

Labs: _____

Therapy: _____

Pharmacy: _____

Visits: _____

Treatments:_____

Date: _____ Name: _____

Specialty: _____ Purpose: _____

Outcome: _____

_____

Conversations: _____

_____

Dr. Instructions: _____

_____

Date: _____ Name: _____

Specialty: _____ Purpose: _____

Outcome: _____

_____

Conversations: _____

_____

Dr. Instructions: _____

_____

Medication Name:	Strength/Dose:	When?
_____	_____	_____
_____	_____	_____
_____	_____	_____

NAME: _____

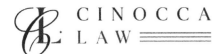

CINOCCA LAW

NAME: _____

DATE: _____ **DAYS POST INJURY:** _____

Body Areas Affected & How

Check any & all body parts affected by the accident:

Head and Neck

- ☐ Head
- ☐ Neck
- ☐ Face
- ☐ Ears
- ☐ Eyes
- ☐ Nose
- ☐ Hair
- ☐ Mouth
- ☐ Jaw
- ☐ Teeth
- ☐ Tongue

Upper Body

- ☐ Shoulders
- ☐ Back
- ☐ Upper Back
- ☐ Lower Back
- ☐ Arms
- ☐ Elbows
- ☐ Hands
- ☐ Wrists
- ☐ Fingers
- ☐ Chest
- ☐ Sternum
- ☐ Torso

Lower Body

- ☐ Hips
- ☐ Bottom
- ☐ Legs
- ☐ Thighs
- ☐ Knees
- ☐ Calves
- ☐ Ankles
- ☐ Feet
- ☐ Toes

Sensory Systems

- ☐ Taste
- ☐ Smell
- ☐ Hearing
- ☐ Sight
- ☐ Throat

Other

- ☐ Mental
- ☐ _____
- ☐ _____
- ☐ _____
- ☐ _____
- ☐ _____
- ☐ _____

Describe the pain in your own words: _____

_____

_____

_____

_____

_____

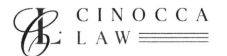

CINOCCA LAW

NAME: _____

DATE: _____ **DAYS POST INJURY:** _____

Body Areas Affected & How

Check any & all body parts affected by the accident:

Head and Neck

- ☐ Head
- ☐ Neck
- ☐ Face
- ☐ Ears
- ☐ Eyes
- ☐ Nose
- ☐ Hair
- ☐ Mouth
- ☐ Jaw
- ☐ Teeth
- ☐ Tongue

Upper Body

- ☐ Shoulders
- ☐ Back
- ☐ Upper Back
- ☐ Lower Back
- ☐ Arms
- ☐ Elbows
- ☐ Hands
- ☐ Wrists
- ☐ Fingers
- ☐ Chest
- ☐ Sternum
- ☐ Torso

Lower Body

- ☐ Hips
- ☐ Bottom
- ☐ Legs
- ☐ Thighs
- ☐ Knees
- ☐ Calves
- ☐ Ankles
- ☐ Feet
- ☐ Toes

Sensory Systems

- ☐ Taste
- ☐ Smell
- ☐ Hearing
- ☐ Sight
- ☐ Throat

Other

- ☐ Mental
- ☐ _____
- ☐ _____
- ☐ _____
- ☐ _____
- ☐ _____
- ☐ _____

Describe the pain in your own words: _____

_____

_____

_____

_____

_____

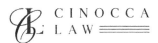

Date: _____   Day: _____

Severity of Pain

Morning: _____

Afternoon: _____

Evening: _____

Middle of Night: _____

Type of Pain   ☐ Throbbing   ☐ Aching   ☐ Stabbing   ☐ _____

Appetite: _____

Sleep: _____

Emotional Well Being

Mood Rating 1-10: _____

Emotional Issues: _____

_____

Nightmares: _____

Fears, Worries, Concerns: _____

_____

Observations

Changes in Symptoms: _____

Side Effects from Medications: _____

Improvements: _____

Deteriorations in Conditions: _____

Medications Taken When & Amount: _____

Limitations on Range of Motion: _____

Impairment of Daily Activities: _____

Help Needed: _____

_____

Help Received: _____

_____

NAME: _____

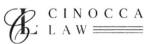

CINOCCA
LAW

Date: _____ Day: _____

Appointments

Drs.: _____

Clinics: _____

Labs: _____

Therapy: _____

Pharmacy: _____

Visits: _____

Treatments: _____

Date: _____   Name: _____

Specialty: _____   Purpose: _____

Outcome: _____

_____

Conversations: _____

_____

Dr. Instructions: _____

_____

Date: _____   Name: _____

Specialty: _____   Purpose: _____

Outcome: _____

_____

Conversations: _____

_____

Dr. Instructions: _____

_____

Medication Name: Strength/Dose: When?

_____   _____   _____

_____   _____   _____

_____   _____   _____

NAME: _____

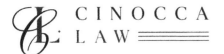

CINOCCA LAW

NAME: _____

DATE: _____ **DAYS POST INJURY:** _____

Body Areas Affected & How

Check any & all body parts affected by the accident:

Head and Neck

☐ Head
☐ Neck
☐ Face
☐ Ears
☐ Eyes
☐ Nose
☐ Hair
☐ Mouth
☐ Jaw
☐ Teeth
☐ Tongue

Upper Body

☐ Shoulders
☐ Back
☐ Upper Back
☐ Lower Back
☐ Arms
☐ Elbows
☐ Hands
☐ Wrists
☐ Fingers
☐ Chest
☐ Sternum
☐ Torso

Lower Body

☐ Hips
☐ Bottom
☐ Legs
☐ Thighs
☐ Knees
☐ Calves
☐ Ankles
☐ Feet
☐ Toes

Sensory Systems

☐ Taste
☐ Smell
☐ Hearing
☐ Sight
☐ Throat

Other

☐ Mental
☐ _____
☐ _____
☐ _____
☐ _____
☐ _____
☐ _____

Describe the pain in your own words: _____

_____

_____

_____

_____

_____

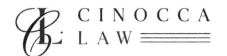

CINOCCA LAW

Personal and Confidential Communication Subject to Attorney Client and Work Product Privilege

NAME: _____

DATE: _____ **DAYS POST INJURY:** _____

Body Areas Affected & How

Check any & all body parts affected by the accident:

Head and Neck
- ☐ Head
- ☐ Neck
- ☐ Face
- ☐ Ears
- ☐ Eyes
- ☐ Nose
- ☐ Hair
- ☐ Mouth
- ☐ Jaw
- ☐ Teeth
- ☐ Tongue

Upper Body
- ☐ Shoulders
- ☐ Back
- ☐ Upper Back
- ☐ Lower Back
- ☐ Arms
- ☐ Elbows
- ☐ Hands
- ☐ Wrists
- ☐ Fingers
- ☐ Chest
- ☐ Sternum
- ☐ Torso

Lower Body
- ☐ Hips
- ☐ Bottom
- ☐ Legs
- ☐ Thighs
- ☐ Knees
- ☐ Calves
- ☐ Ankles
- ☐ Feet
- ☐ Toes

Sensory Systems
- ☐ Taste
- ☐ Smell
- ☐ Hearing
- ☐ Sight
- ☐ Throat

Other
- ☐ Mental
- ☐ _____
- ☐ _____
- ☐ _____
- ☐ _____
- ☐ _____

Describe the pain in your own words: _____

_____

_____

_____

_____

_____

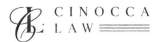

Date: _____ Day: _____

Severity of Pain

Morning: _____

Afternoon: _____

Evening: _____

Middle of Night: _____

Type of Pain   ☐ Throbbing   ☐ Aching   ☐ Stabbing   ☐ _____

Appetite: _____

Sleep: _____

Emotional Well Being

Mood Rating 1-10: _____

Emotional Issues: _____

_____

Nightmares: _____

Fears, Worries, Concerns: _____

_____

Observations

Changes in Symptoms: _____

Side Effects from Medications: _____

Improvements: _____

Deteriorations in Conditions: _____

Medications Taken When & Amount: _____

Limitations on Range of Motion: _____

Impairment of Daily Activities: _____

Help Needed: _____

_____

Help Received: _____

_____

NAME: _____

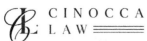

Date: _____ Day: _____

Appointments

Drs.: _____

Clinics: _____

Labs: _____

Therapy: _____

Pharmacy: _____

Visits: _____

Treatments: _____

Date: _____ Name: _____

Specialty: _____ Purpose: _____

Outcome: _____
_____

Conversations: _____
_____

Dr. Instructions: _____
_____

Date: _____ Name: _____

Specialty: _____ Purpose: _____

Outcome: _____
_____

Conversations: _____
_____

Dr. Instructions: _____
_____

Medication Name:	Strength/Dose:	When?
_____	_____	_____
_____	_____	_____
_____	_____	_____

NAME: _____

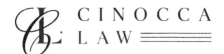

NAME: _____

DATE: _____ **DAYS POST INJURY:** _____

Body Areas Affected & How

Check any & all body parts affected by the accident:

Head and Neck

☐ Head
☐ Neck
☐ Face
☐ Ears
☐ Eyes
☐ Nose
☐ Hair
☐ Mouth
☐ Jaw
☐ Teeth
☐ Tongue

Upper Body

☐ Shoulders
☐ Back
☐ Upper Back
☐ Lower Back
☐ Arms
☐ Elbows
☐ Hands
☐ Wrists
☐ Fingers
☐ Chest
☐ Sternum
☐ Torso

Lower Body

☐ Hips
☐ Bottom
☐ Legs
☐ Thighs
☐ Knees
☐ Calves
☐ Ankles
☐ Feet
☐ Toes

Sensory Systems

☐ Taste
☐ Smell
☐ Hearing
☐ Sight
☐ Throat

Other

☐ Mental
☐ _____
☐ _____
☐ _____
☐ _____
☐ _____
☐ _____

Describe the pain in your own words: _____

_____

_____

_____

_____

_____

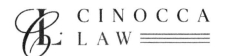

NAME: _____

DATE: _____ **DAYS POST INJURY:** _____

Body Areas Affected & How

Check any & all body parts affected by the accident:

Head and Neck

- ☐ Head
- ☐ Neck
- ☐ Face
- ☐ Ears
- ☐ Eyes
- ☐ Nose
- ☐ Hair
- ☐ Mouth
- ☐ Jaw
- ☐ Teeth
- ☐ Tongue

Upper Body

- ☐ Shoulders
- ☐ Back
- ☐ Upper Back
- ☐ Lower Back
- ☐ Arms
- ☐ Elbows
- ☐ Hands
- ☐ Wrists
- ☐ Fingers
- ☐ Chest
- ☐ Sternum
- ☐ Torso

Lower Body

- ☐ Hips
- ☐ Bottom
- ☐ Legs
- ☐ Thighs
- ☐ Knees
- ☐ Calves
- ☐ Ankles
- ☐ Feet
- ☐ Toes

Sensory Systems

- ☐ Taste
- ☐ Smell
- ☐ Hearing
- ☐ Sight
- ☐ Throat

Other

- ☐ Mental
- ☐ _____
- ☐ _____
- ☐ _____
- ☐ _____
- ☐ _____
- ☐ _____

Describe the pain in your own words: _____

_____

_____

_____

_____

_____

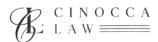

Date: _____   Day: _____

Severity of Pain

Morning: _____

Afternoon: _____

Evening: _____

Middle of Night: _____

Type of Pain   ☐ Throbbing   ☐ Aching   ☐ Stabbing   ☐ _____

Appetite: _____

Sleep: _____

Emotional Well Being

Mood Rating 1-10: _____

Emotional Issues: _____

_____

Nightmares: _____

Fears, Worries, Concerns: _____

_____

Observations

Changes in Symptoms: _____

Side Effects from Medications: _____

Improvements: _____

Deteriorations in Conditions: _____

Medications Taken When & Amount: _____

Limitations on Range of Motion: _____

Impairment of Daily Activities: _____

Help Needed: _____

_____

Help Received: _____

_____

NAME: _____

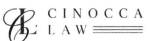

Date: _____ Day: _____

Appointments

Drs.: _____

Clinics: _____

Labs: _____

Therapy: _____

Pharmacy: _____

Visits: _____

Treatments: _____

Date: _____ Name: _____

Specialty: _____ Purpose: _____

Outcome: _____

_____

Conversations: _____

_____

Dr. Instructions: _____

_____

Date: _____ Name: _____

Specialty: _____ Purpose: _____

Outcome: _____

_____

Conversations: _____

_____

Dr. Instructions: _____

_____

Medication Name:	Strength/Dose:	When?
_____	_____	_____
_____	_____	_____
_____	_____	_____

NAME: _____

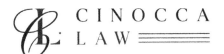

Personal and Confidential Communication Subject to
Attorney Client and Work Product Privilege

NAME: _____

DATE: _____ **DAYS POST INJURY:** _____

Body Areas Affected & How

Check any & all body parts affected by the accident:

Head and Neck

☐ Head
☐ Neck
☐ Face
☐ Ears
☐ Eyes
☐ Nose
☐ Hair
☐ Mouth
☐ Jaw
☐ Teeth
☐ Tongue

Upper Body

☐ Shoulders
☐ Back
☐ Upper Back
☐ Lower Back
☐ Arms
☐ Elbows
☐ Hands
☐ Wrists
☐ Fingers
☐ Chest
☐ Sternum
☐ Torso

Lower Body

☐ Hips
☐ Bottom
☐ Legs
☐ Thighs
☐ Knees
☐ Calves
☐ Ankles
☐ Feet
☐ Toes

Sensory Systems

☐ Taste
☐ Smell
☐ Hearing
☐ Sight
☐ Throat

Other

☐ Mental
☐ _____
☐ _____
☐ _____
☐ _____
☐ _____
☐ _____

Describe the pain in your own words: _____

_____

_____

_____

_____

_____

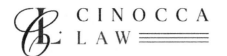

CINOCCA LAW

Personal and Confidential Communication Subject to Attorney Client and Work Product Privilege

NAME: _____

DATE: _____ **DAYS POST INJURY:** _____

Body Areas Affected & How

Check any & all body parts affected by the accident:

Head and Neck

- ☐ Head
- ☐ Neck
- ☐ Face
- ☐ Ears
- ☐ Eyes
- ☐ Nose
- ☐ Hair
- ☐ Mouth
- ☐ Jaw
- ☐ Teeth
- ☐ Tongue

Upper Body

- ☐ Shoulders
- ☐ Back
- ☐ Upper Back
- ☐ Lower Back
- ☐ Arms
- ☐ Elbows
- ☐ Hands
- ☐ Wrists
- ☐ Fingers
- ☐ Chest
- ☐ Sternum
- ☐ Torso

Lower Body

- ☐ Hips
- ☐ Bottom
- ☐ Legs
- ☐ Thighs
- ☐ Knees
- ☐ Calves
- ☐ Ankles
- ☐ Feet
- ☐ Toes

Sensory Systems

- ☐ Taste
- ☐ Smell
- ☐ Hearing
- ☐ Sight
- ☐ Throat

Other

- ☐ Mental
- ☐ _____
- ☐ _____
- ☐ _____
- ☐ _____
- ☐ _____
- ☐ _____

Describe the pain in your own words: _____

_____

_____

_____

_____

_____

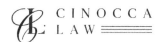

Date: _____   Day: _____

Severity of Pain

Morning: _____

Afternoon: _____

Evening: _____

Middle of Night: _____

Type of Pain   ☐ Throbbing   ☐ Aching   ☐ Stabbing   ☐ _____

Appetite: _____

Sleep: _____

Emotional Well Being

Mood Rating 1-10: _____

Emotional Issues: _____

_____

Nightmares: _____

Fears, Worries, Concerns: _____

_____

Observations

Changes in Symptoms: _____

Side Effects from Medications: _____

Improvements: _____

Deteriorations in Conditions: _____

Medications Taken When & Amount: _____

Limitations on Range of Motion: _____

Impairment of Daily Activities: _____

Help Needed: _____

_____

Help Received: _____

_____

NAME: _____

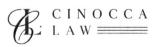

Date: _____   Day: _____

Appointments

Drs.: _____

Clinics: _____

Labs: _____

Therapy: _____

Pharmacy: _____

Visits: _____

Treatments: _____

Date: _____   Name: _____

Specialty: _____   Purpose: _____

Outcome: _____

_____

Conversations: _____

_____

Dr. Instructions: _____

_____

Date: _____   Name: _____

Specialty: _____   Purpose: _____

Outcome: _____

_____

Conversations: _____

_____

Dr. Instructions: _____

_____

Medication Name:	Strength/Dose:	When?
_____	_____	_____
_____	_____	_____
_____	_____	_____

NAME: _____

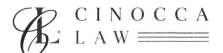

NAME: _____

DATE: _____ **DAYS POST INJURY:** _____

Body Areas Affected & How

Check any & all body parts affected by the accident:

Head and Neck

- ☐ Head
- ☐ Neck
- ☐ Face
- ☐ Ears
- ☐ Eyes
- ☐ Nose
- ☐ Hair
- ☐ Mouth
- ☐ Jaw
- ☐ Teeth
- ☐ Tongue

Upper Body

- ☐ Shoulders
- ☐ Back
- ☐ Upper Back
- ☐ Lower Back
- ☐ Arms
- ☐ Elbows
- ☐ Hands
- ☐ Wrists
- ☐ Fingers
- ☐ Chest
- ☐ Sternum
- ☐ Torso

Lower Body

- ☐ Hips
- ☐ Bottom
- ☐ Legs
- ☐ Thighs
- ☐ Knees
- ☐ Calves
- ☐ Ankles
- ☐ Feet
- ☐ Toes

Sensory Systems

- ☐ Taste
- ☐ Smell
- ☐ Hearing
- ☐ Sight
- ☐ Throat

Other

- ☐ Mental
- ☐ _____
- ☐ _____
- ☐ _____
- ☐ _____
- ☐ _____
- ☐ _____

Describe the pain in your own words: _____

_____

_____

_____

_____

_____

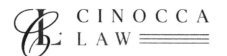

NAME: _____

DATE: _____ **DAYS POST INJURY:** _____

Body Areas Affected & How

Check any & all body parts affected by the accident:

Head and Neck
- ☐ Head
- ☐ Neck
- ☐ Face
- ☐ Ears
- ☐ Eyes
- ☐ Nose
- ☐ Hair
- ☐ Mouth
- ☐ Jaw
- ☐ Teeth
- ☐ Tongue

Upper Body
- ☐ Shoulders
- ☐ Back
- ☐ Upper Back
- ☐ Lower Back
- ☐ Arms
- ☐ Elbows
- ☐ Hands
- ☐ Wrists
- ☐ Fingers
- ☐ Chest
- ☐ Sternum
- ☐ Torso

Lower Body
- ☐ Hips
- ☐ Bottom
- ☐ Legs
- ☐ Thighs
- ☐ Knees
- ☐ Calves
- ☐ Ankles
- ☐ Feet
- ☐ Toes

Sensory Systems
- ☐ Taste
- ☐ Smell
- ☐ Hearing
- ☐ Sight
- ☐ Throat

Other
- ☐ Mental
- ☐ _____
- ☐ _____
- ☐ _____
- ☐ _____
- ☐ _____
- ☐ _____

Describe the pain in your own words: _____

_____

_____

_____

_____

_____

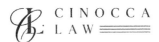

Date: _____ Day: _____

Severity of Pain

Morning: _____

Afternoon: _____

Evening: _____

Middle of Night: _____

Type of Pain ☐ Throbbing ☐ Aching ☐ Stabbing ☐ _____

Appetite: _____

Sleep: _____

Emotional Well Being

Mood Rating 1-10: _____

Emotional Issues: _____

_____

Nightmares: _____

Fears, Worries, Concerns: _____

_____

Observations

Changes in Symptoms: _____

Side Effects from Medications: _____

Improvements: _____

Deteriorations in Conditions: _____

Medications Taken When & Amount: _____

Limitations on Range of Motion: _____

Impairment of Daily Activities: _____

Help Needed: _____

_____

Help Received: _____

_____

NAME: _____

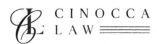

Date: _____ Day: _____

Appointments

Drs.: _____

Clinics: _____

Labs: _____

Therapy: _____

Pharmacy: _____

Visits: _____

Treatments: _____

Date: _____ Name: _____

Specialty: _____ Purpose: _____

Outcome: _____

_____

Conversations: _____

_____

Dr. Instructions: _____

_____

Date: _____ Name: _____

Specialty: _____ Purpose: _____

Outcome: _____

_____

Conversations: _____

_____

Dr. Instructions: _____

_____

Medication Name:	Strength/Dose:	When?
_____	_____	_____
_____	_____	_____
_____	_____	_____

NAME: _____

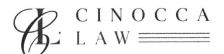

NAME: _____

DATE: _____ **DAYS POST INJURY:** _____

Body Areas Affected & How

Check any & all body parts affected by the accident:

Head and Neck

- ☐ Head
- ☐ Neck
- ☐ Face
- ☐ Ears
- ☐ Eyes
- ☐ Nose
- ☐ Hair
- ☐ Mouth
- ☐ Jaw
- ☐ Teeth
- ☐ Tongue

Upper Body

- ☐ Shoulders
- ☐ Back
- ☐ Upper Back
- ☐ Lower Back
- ☐ Arms
- ☐ Elbows
- ☐ Hands
- ☐ Wrists
- ☐ Fingers
- ☐ Chest
- ☐ Sternum
- ☐ Torso

Lower Body

- ☐ Hips
- ☐ Bottom
- ☐ Legs
- ☐ Thighs
- ☐ Knees
- ☐ Calves
- ☐ Ankles
- ☐ Feet
- ☐ Toes

Sensory Systems

- ☐ Taste
- ☐ Smell
- ☐ Hearing
- ☐ Sight
- ☐ Throat

Other

- ☐ Mental
- ☐ _____
- ☐ _____
- ☐ _____
- ☐ _____
- ☐ _____
- ☐ _____

Describe the pain in your own words: _____

_____

_____

_____

_____

_____

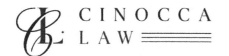 C I N O C C A
L A W

Personal and Confidential Communication Subject to Attorney Client and Work Product Privilege

NAME: _____

DATE: _____ **DAYS POST INJURY:** _____

Body Areas Affected & How

Check any & all body parts affected by the accident:

Head and Neck
☐ Head
☐ Neck
☐ Face
☐ Ears
☐ Eyes
☐ Nose
☐ Hair
☐ Mouth
☐ Jaw
☐ Teeth
☐ Tongue

Upper Body
☐ Shoulders
☐ Back
☐ Upper Back
☐ Lower Back
☐ Arms
☐ Elbows
☐ Hands
☐ Wrists
☐ Fingers
☐ Chest
☐ Sternum
☐ Torso

Lower Body
☐ Hips
☐ Bottom
☐ Legs
☐ Thighs
☐ Knees
☐ Calves
☐ Ankles
☐ Feet
☐ Toes

Sensory Systems
☐ Taste
☐ Smell
☐ Hearing
☐ Sight
☐ Throat

Other
☐ Mental
☐ _____
☐ _____
☐ _____
☐ _____
☐ _____
☐ _____

Describe the pain in your own words: _____

_____

_____

_____

_____

_____

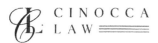

Date: _____   Day: _____

Severity of Pain

Morning: _____

Afternoon: _____

Evening: _____

Middle of Night: _____

Type of Pain   ☐ Throbbing   ☐ Aching   ☐ Stabbing   ☐ _____

Appetite: _____

Sleep: _____

Emotional Well Being

Mood Rating 1-10: _____

Emotional Issues: _____

_____

Nightmares: _____

Fears, Worries, Concerns: _____

_____

Observations

Changes in Symptoms: _____

Side Effects from Medications: _____

Improvements: _____

Deteriorations in Conditions: _____

Medications Taken When & Amount: _____

Limitations on Range of Motion: _____

Impairment of Daily Activities: _____

Help Needed: _____

_____

Help Received: _____

_____

NAME: _____

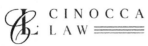

Date: _____ Day: _____

Appointments

Drs.: _____

Clinics: _____

Labs: _____

Therapy: _____

Pharmacy: _____

Visits: _____

Treatments: _____

Date: _____ Name: _____

Specialty: _____ Purpose: _____

Outcome: _____

_____

Conversations: _____

_____

Dr. Instructions: _____

_____

Date: _____ Name: _____

Specialty: _____ Purpose: _____

Outcome: _____

_____

Conversations: _____

_____

Dr. Instructions: _____

_____

Medication Name:	Strength/Dose:	When?
_____	_____	_____
_____	_____	_____
_____	_____	_____

NAME: _____

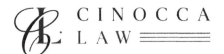

Personal and Confidential Communication Subject to Attorney Client and Work Product Privilege

NAME: _____

DATE: _____   **DAYS POST INJURY:** _____

Body Areas Affected & How

Check any & all body parts affected by the accident:

Head and Neck

☐ Head
☐ Neck
☐ Face
☐ Ears
☐ Eyes
☐ Nose
☐ Hair
☐ Mouth
☐ Jaw
☐ Teeth
☐ Tongue

Upper Body

☐ Shoulders
☐ Back
☐ Upper Back
☐ Lower Back
☐ Arms
☐ Elbows
☐ Hands
☐ Wrists
☐ Fingers
☐ Chest
☐ Sternum
☐ Torso

Lower Body

☐ Hips
☐ Bottom
☐ Legs
☐ Thighs
☐ Knees
☐ Calves
☐ Ankles
☐ Feet
☐ Toes

Sensory Systems

☐ Taste
☐ Smell
☐ Hearing
☐ Sight
☐ Throat

Other

☐ Mental
☐ _____
☐ _____
☐ _____
☐ _____
☐ _____
☐ _____

Describe the pain in your own words: _____

_____

_____

_____

_____

_____

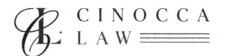

CINOCCA LAW

Personal and Confidential Communication Subject to Attorney Client and Work Product Privilege

NAME: _____

DATE: _____ DAYS POST INJURY: _____

Body Areas Affected & How

Check any & all body parts affected by the accident:

Head and Neck
- ☐ Head
- ☐ Neck
- ☐ Face
- ☐ Ears
- ☐ Eyes
- ☐ Nose
- ☐ Hair
- ☐ Mouth
- ☐ Jaw
- ☐ Teeth
- ☐ Tongue

Upper Body
- ☐ Shoulders
- ☐ Back
- ☐ Upper Back
- ☐ Lower Back
- ☐ Arms
- ☐ Elbows
- ☐ Hands
- ☐ Wrists
- ☐ Fingers
- ☐ Chest
- ☐ Sternum
- ☐ Torso

Lower Body
- ☐ Hips
- ☐ Bottom
- ☐ Legs
- ☐ Thighs
- ☐ Knees
- ☐ Calves
- ☐ Ankles
- ☐ Feet
- ☐ Toes

Sensory Systems
- ☐ Taste
- ☐ Smell
- ☐ Hearing
- ☐ Sight
- ☐ Throat

Other
- ☐ Mental
- ☐ _____
- ☐ _____
- ☐ _____
- ☐ _____
- ☐ _____
- ☐ _____

Describe the pain in your own words: _____

_____

_____

_____

_____

_____

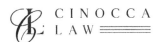

Date: _____   Day: _____

Severity of Pain

Morning: _____

Afternoon: _____

Evening: _____

Middle of Night: _____

Type of Pain   ☐ Throbbing   ☐ Aching   ☐ Stabbing   ☐ _____

Appetite: _____

Sleep: _____

Emotional Well Being

Mood Rating 1-10: _____

Emotional Issues: _____

_____

Nightmares: _____

Fears, Worries, Concerns: _____

_____

Observations

Changes in Symptoms: _____

Side Effects from Medications: _____

Improvements: _____

Deteriorations in Conditions: _____

Medications Taken When & Amount: _____

Limitations on Range of Motion: _____

Impairment of Daily Activities: _____

Help Needed: _____

_____

Help Received: _____

_____

NAME: _____

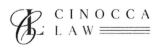

Appointments

Drs.: _____

Clinics: _____

Labs: _____

Therapy: _____

Pharmacy: _____

Visits: _____

Treatments: _____

Date: _____ Name: _____

Specialty: _____ Purpose: _____

Outcome: _____

_____

Conversations: _____

_____

Dr. Instructions: _____

_____

Date: _____ Name: _____

Specialty: _____ Purpose: _____

Outcome: _____

_____

Conversations: _____

_____

Dr. Instructions: _____

_____

Medication Name:	Strength/Dose:	When?
_____	_____	_____
_____	_____	_____
_____	_____	_____

NAME: _____

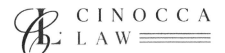

NAME: _____

DATE: _____ **DAYS POST INJURY:** _____

Body Areas Affected & How

Check any & all body parts affected by the accident:

Head and Neck

☐ Head
☐ Neck
☐ Face
☐ Ears
☐ Eyes
☐ Nose
☐ Hair
☐ Mouth
☐ Jaw
☐ Teeth
☐ Tongue

Upper Body

☐ Shoulders
☐ Back
☐ Upper Back
☐ Lower Back
☐ Arms
☐ Elbows
☐ Hands
☐ Wrists
☐ Fingers
☐ Chest
☐ Sternum
☐ Torso

Lower Body

☐ Hips
☐ Bottom
☐ Legs
☐ Thighs
☐ Knees
☐ Calves
☐ Ankles
☐ Feet
☐ Toes

Sensory Systems

☐ Taste
☐ Smell
☐ Hearing
☐ Sight
☐ Throat

Other

☐ Mental
☐ _____
☐ _____
☐ _____
☐ _____
☐ _____
☐ _____

Describe the pain in your own words: _____

_____

_____

_____

_____

_____

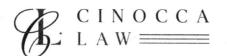

NAME: _____

DATE: _____ **DAYS POST INJURY:** _____

Body Areas Affected & How

Check any & all body parts affected by the accident:

Head and Neck
- ☐ Head
- ☐ Neck
- ☐ Face
- ☐ Ears
- ☐ Eyes
- ☐ Nose
- ☐ Hair
- ☐ Mouth
- ☐ Jaw
- ☐ Teeth
- ☐ Tongue

Upper Body
- ☐ Shoulders
- ☐ Back
- ☐ Upper Back
- ☐ Lower Back
- ☐ Arms
- ☐ Elbows
- ☐ Hands
- ☐ Wrists
- ☐ Fingers
- ☐ Chest
- ☐ Sternum
- ☐ Torso

Lower Body
- ☐ Hips
- ☐ Bottom
- ☐ Legs
- ☐ Thighs
- ☐ Knees
- ☐ Calves
- ☐ Ankles
- ☐ Feet
- ☐ Toes

Sensory Systems
- ☐ Taste
- ☐ Smell
- ☐ Hearing
- ☐ Sight
- ☐ Throat

Other
- ☐ Mental
- ☐ _____
- ☐ _____
- ☐ _____
- ☐ _____
- ☐ _____
- ☐ _____

Describe the pain in your own words: _____

_____

_____

_____

_____

_____

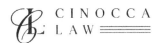

Date: _____   Day: _____

Severity of Pain

Morning: _____

Afternoon: _____

Evening: _____

Middle of Night: _____

Type of Pain   ☐ Throbbing   ☐ Aching   ☐ Stabbing   ☐ _____ _____

Appetite: _____

Sleep: _____

Emotional Well Being

Mood Rating 1-10: _____

Emotional Issues: _____

_____

Nightmares: _____

Fears, Worries, Concerns: _____

_____

Observations

Changes in Symptoms: _____

Side Effects from Medications: _____

Improvements: _____

Deteriorations in Conditions: _____

Medications Taken When & Amount: _____

Limitations on Range of Motion: _____

Impairment of Daily Activities: _____

Help Needed: _____

_____

Help Received: _____

_____

NAME: _____

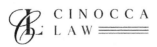

Date: _____ Day: _____

Appointments

Drs.: _____

Clinics: _____

Labs: _____

Therapy: _____

Pharmacy: _____

Visits: _____

Treatments: _____

Date: _____ Name: _____

Specialty: _____ Purpose: _____

Outcome: _____

_____

Conversations: _____

_____

Dr. Instructions: _____

_____

Date: _____ Name: _____

Specialty: _____ Purpose: _____

Outcome: _____

_____

Conversations: _____

_____

Dr. Instructions: _____

_____

Medication Name: Strength/Dose: When?

_____   _____   _____

_____   _____   _____

_____   _____   _____

NAME: _____

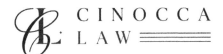

NAME: _____

DATE: _____ **DAYS POST INJURY:** _____

Body Areas Affected & How

Check any & all body parts affected by the accident:

Head and Neck

- ☐ Head
- ☐ Neck
- ☐ Face
- ☐ Ears
- ☐ Eyes
- ☐ Nose
- ☐ Hair
- ☐ Mouth
- ☐ Jaw
- ☐ Teeth
- ☐ Tongue

Upper Body

- ☐ Shoulders
- ☐ Back
- ☐ Upper Back
- ☐ Lower Back
- ☐ Arms
- ☐ Elbows
- ☐ Hands
- ☐ Wrists
- ☐ Fingers
- ☐ Chest
- ☐ Sternum
- ☐ Torso

Lower Body

- ☐ Hips
- ☐ Bottom
- ☐ Legs
- ☐ Thighs
- ☐ Knees
- ☐ Calves
- ☐ Ankles
- ☐ Feet
- ☐ Toes

Sensory Systems

- ☐ Taste
- ☐ Smell
- ☐ Hearing
- ☐ Sight
- ☐ Throat

Other

- ☐ Mental
- ☐ _____
- ☐ _____
- ☐ _____
- ☐ _____
- ☐ _____
- ☐ _____

Describe the pain in your own words: _____

_____

_____

_____

_____

_____

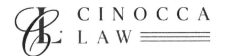

NAME: _____

DATE: _____   **DAYS POST INJURY:** _____

Body Areas Affected & How

Check any & all body parts affected by the accident:

Head and Neck

- ☐ Head
- ☐ Neck
- ☐ Face
- ☐ Ears
- ☐ Eyes
- ☐ Nose
- ☐ Hair
- ☐ Mouth
- ☐ Jaw
- ☐ Teeth
- ☐ Tongue

Upper Body

- ☐ Shoulders
- ☐ Back
- ☐ Upper Back
- ☐ Lower Back
- ☐ Arms
- ☐ Elbows
- ☐ Hands
- ☐ Wrists
- ☐ Fingers
- ☐ Chest
- ☐ Sternum
- ☐ Torso

Lower Body

- ☐ Hips
- ☐ Bottom
- ☐ Legs
- ☐ Thighs
- ☐ Knees
- ☐ Calves
- ☐ Ankles
- ☐ Feet
- ☐ Toes

Sensory Systems

- ☐ Taste
- ☐ Smell
- ☐ Hearing
- ☐ Sight
- ☐ Throat

Other

- ☐ Mental
- ☐ _____
- ☐ _____
- ☐ _____
- ☐ _____
- ☐ _____
- ☐ _____

Describe the pain in your own words: _____

_____

_____

_____

_____

_____

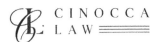

Date: _____   Day: _____

Severity of Pain

Morning: _____

Afternoon: _____

Evening: _____

Middle of Night: _____

Type of Pain   ☐ Throbbing   ☐ Aching   ☐ Stabbing   ☐ _____

Appetite: _____

Sleep: _____

Emotional Well Being

Mood Rating 1-10: _____

Emotional Issues: _____

_____

Nightmares: _____

Fears, Worries, Concerns: _____

_____

Observations

Changes in Symptoms: _____

Side Effects from Medications: _____

Improvements: _____

Deteriorations in Conditions: _____

Medications Taken When & Amount: _____

Limitations on Range of Motion: _____

Impairment of Daily Activities: _____

Help Needed: _____

_____

Help Received: _____

_____

NAME: _____

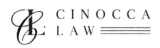

Date: _____ Day: _____

Appointments

Drs.: _____

Clinics: _____

Labs: _____

Therapy: _____

Pharmacy: _____

Visits: _____

Treatments: _____

Date: _____ Name: _____

Specialty: _____ Purpose: _____

Outcome: _____

_____

Conversations: _____

_____

Dr. Instructions: _____

_____

Date: _____ Name: _____

Specialty: _____ Purpose: _____

Outcome: _____

_____

Conversations: _____

_____

Dr. Instructions: _____

_____

Medication Name:	Strength/Dose:	When?
_____	_____	_____
_____	_____	_____
_____	_____	_____

NAME: _____

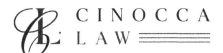

CINOCCA LAW

Personal and Confidential Communication Subject to Attorney Client and Work Product Privilege

NAME: _____

DATE: _____ **DAYS POST INJURY:** _____

Body Areas Affected & How

Check any & all body parts affected by the accident:

Head and Neck

- ☐ Head
- ☐ Neck
- ☐ Face
- ☐ Ears
- ☐ Eyes
- ☐ Nose
- ☐ Hair
- ☐ Mouth
- ☐ Jaw
- ☐ Teeth
- ☐ Tongue

Upper Body

- ☐ Shoulders
- ☐ Back
- ☐ Upper Back
- ☐ Lower Back
- ☐ Arms
- ☐ Elbows
- ☐ Hands
- ☐ Wrists
- ☐ Fingers
- ☐ Chest
- ☐ Sternum
- ☐ Torso

Lower Body

- ☐ Hips
- ☐ Bottom
- ☐ Legs
- ☐ Thighs
- ☐ Knees
- ☐ Calves
- ☐ Ankles
- ☐ Feet
- ☐ Toes

Sensory Systems

- ☐ Taste
- ☐ Smell
- ☐ Hearing
- ☐ Sight
- ☐ Throat

Other

- ☐ Mental
- ☐ _____
- ☐ _____
- ☐ _____
- ☐ _____
- ☐ _____
- ☐ _____

Describe the pain in your own words: _____

_____

_____

_____

_____

_____

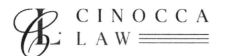

NAME: _____

DATE: _____   DAYS POST INJURY: _____

Body Areas Affected & How

Check any & all body parts affected by the accident:

Head and Neck
- ☐ Head
- ☐ Neck
- ☐ Face
- ☐ Ears
- ☐ Eyes
- ☐ Nose
- ☐ Hair
- ☐ Mouth
- ☐ Jaw
- ☐ Teeth
- ☐ Tongue

Upper Body
- ☐ Shoulders
- ☐ Back
- ☐ Upper Back
- ☐ Lower Back
- ☐ Arms
- ☐ Elbows
- ☐ Hands
- ☐ Wrists
- ☐ Fingers
- ☐ Chest
- ☐ Sternum
- ☐ Torso

Lower Body
- ☐ Hips
- ☐ Bottom
- ☐ Legs
- ☐ Thighs
- ☐ Knees
- ☐ Calves
- ☐ Ankles
- ☐ Feet
- ☐ Toes

Sensory Systems
- ☐ Taste
- ☐ Smell
- ☐ Hearing
- ☐ Sight
- ☐ Throat

Other
- ☐ Mental
- ☐ _____
- ☐ _____
- ☐ _____
- ☐ _____
- ☐ _____
- ☐ _____

Describe the pain in your own words: _____

_____

_____

_____

_____

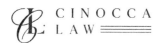

Date: _____   Day: _____

Severity of Pain

Morning: _____

Afternoon: _____

Evening: _____

Middle of Night: _____

Type of Pain   ☐ Throbbing   ☐ Aching   ☐ Stabbing   ☐ _____

Appetite: _____

Sleep: _____

Emotional Well Being

Mood Rating 1-10: _____

Emotional Issues: _____

_____

Nightmares: _____

Fears, Worries, Concerns: _____

_____

Observations

Changes in Symptoms: _____

Side Effects from Medications: _____

Improvements: _____

Deteriorations in Conditions: _____

Medications Taken When & Amount: _____

Limitations on Range of Motion: _____

Impairment of Daily Activities: _____

Help Needed: _____

_____

Help Received: _____

_____

NAME: _____

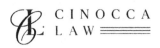
CINOCCA
LAW ≡≡≡

Date: _____   Day: _____

Appointments

Drs.: _____

Clinics: _____

Labs: _____

Therapy: _____

Pharmacy: _____

Visits: _____

Treatments: _____

Date: _____   Name: _____

Specialty: _____   Purpose: _____

Outcome: _____

_____

Conversations: _____

_____

Dr. Instructions: _____

_____

Date: _____   Name: _____

Specialty: _____   Purpose: _____

Outcome: _____

_____

Conversations: _____

_____

Dr. Instructions: _____

_____

Medication Name:	Strength/Dose:	When?
_____	_____	_____
_____	_____	_____
_____	_____	_____

NAME: _____

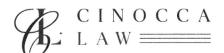

NAME: _____

DATE: _____ **DAYS POST INJURY:** _____

Body Areas Affected & How

Check any & all body parts affected by the accident:

Head and Neck

- ☐ Head
- ☐ Neck
- ☐ Face
- ☐ Ears
- ☐ Eyes
- ☐ Nose
- ☐ Hair
- ☐ Mouth
- ☐ Jaw
- ☐ Teeth
- ☐ Tongue

Upper Body

- ☐ Shoulders
- ☐ Back
- ☐ Upper Back
- ☐ Lower Back
- ☐ Arms
- ☐ Elbows
- ☐ Hands
- ☐ Wrists
- ☐ Fingers
- ☐ Chest
- ☐ Sternum
- ☐ Torso

Lower Body

- ☐ Hips
- ☐ Bottom
- ☐ Legs
- ☐ Thighs
- ☐ Knees
- ☐ Calves
- ☐ Ankles
- ☐ Feet
- ☐ Toes

Sensory Systems

- ☐ Taste
- ☐ Smell
- ☐ Hearing
- ☐ Sight
- ☐ Throat

Other

- ☐ Mental
- ☐ _____
- ☐ _____
- ☐ _____
- ☐ _____
- ☐ _____
- ☐ _____

Describe the pain in your own words: _____

_____

_____

_____

_____

_____

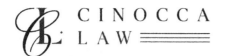

Personal and Confidential Communication Subject to Attorney Client and Work Product Privilege

NAME: _____

DATE: _____   DAYS POST INJURY: _____

Body Areas Affected & How

Check any & all body parts affected by the accident:

Head and Neck
- ☐ Head
- ☐ Neck
- ☐ Face
- ☐ Ears
- ☐ Eyes
- ☐ Nose
- ☐ Hair
- ☐ Mouth
- ☐ Jaw
- ☐ Teeth
- ☐ Tongue

Upper Body
- ☐ Shoulders
- ☐ Back
- ☐ Upper Back
- ☐ Lower Back
- ☐ Arms
- ☐ Elbows
- ☐ Hands
- ☐ Wrists
- ☐ Fingers
- ☐ Chest
- ☐ Sternum
- ☐ Torso

Lower Body
- ☐ Hips
- ☐ Bottom
- ☐ Legs
- ☐ Thighs
- ☐ Knees
- ☐ Calves
- ☐ Ankles
- ☐ Feet
- ☐ Toes

Sensory Systems
- ☐ Taste
- ☐ Smell
- ☐ Hearing
- ☐ Sight
- ☐ Throat

Other
- ☐ Mental
- ☐ _____
- ☐ _____
- ☐ _____
- ☐ _____
- ☐ _____
- ☐ _____

Describe the pain in your own words: _____

_____

_____

_____

_____

_____

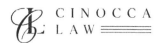

Date: _____   Day: _____

Severity of Pain

Morning: _____

Afternoon: _____

Evening: _____

Middle of Night: _____

Type of Pain   ☐ Throbbing   ☐ Aching   ☐ Stabbing   ☐ _____

Appetite: _____

Sleep: _____

Emotional Well Being

Mood Rating 1-10: _____

Emotional Issues: _____

_____

Nightmares: _____

Fears, Worries, Concerns: _____

_____

Observations

Changes in Symptoms: _____

Side Effects from Medications: _____

Improvements: _____

Deteriorations in Conditions: _____

Medications Taken When & Amount: _____

Limitations on Range of Motion: _____

Impairment of Daily Activities: _____

Help Needed: _____

_____

Help Received: _____

_____

NAME: _____

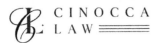

Date: _____ Day: _____

Appointments

Drs.: _____

Clinics: _____

Labs: _____

Therapy: _____

Pharmacy: _____

Visits: _____

Treatments: _____

Date: _____ Name: _____

Specialty: _____ Purpose: _____

Outcome: _____

_____

Conversations: _____

_____

Dr. Instructions: _____

_____

Date: _____ Name: _____

Specialty: _____ Purpose: _____

Outcome: _____

_____

Conversations: _____

_____

Dr. Instructions: _____

_____

Medication Name:	Strength/Dose:	When?
_____	_____	_____
_____	_____	_____
_____	_____	_____

NAME: _____

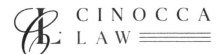

NAME: _____

DATE: _____ DAYS POST INJURY: _____

Body Areas Affected & How

Check any & all body parts affected by the accident:

Head and Neck

- ☐ Head
- ☐ Neck
- ☐ Face
- ☐ Ears
- ☐ Eyes
- ☐ Nose
- ☐ Hair
- ☐ Mouth
- ☐ Jaw
- ☐ Teeth
- ☐ Tongue

Upper Body

- ☐ Shoulders
- ☐ Back
- ☐ Upper Back
- ☐ Lower Back
- ☐ Arms
- ☐ Elbows
- ☐ Hands
- ☐ Wrists
- ☐ Fingers
- ☐ Chest
- ☐ Sternum
- ☐ Torso

Lower Body

- ☐ Hips
- ☐ Bottom
- ☐ Legs
- ☐ Thighs
- ☐ Knees
- ☐ Calves
- ☐ Ankles
- ☐ Feet
- ☐ Toes

Sensory Systems

- ☐ Taste
- ☐ Smell
- ☐ Hearing
- ☐ Sight
- ☐ Throat

Other

- ☐ Mental
- ☐ _____
- ☐ _____
- ☐ _____
- ☐ _____
- ☐ _____
- ☐ _____

Describe the pain in your own words: _____

_____

_____

_____

_____

_____

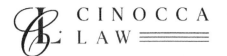

NAME: _____

DATE: _____ **DAYS POST INJURY:** _____

Body Areas Affected & How

Check any & all body parts affected by the accident:

Head and Neck
- ☐ Head
- ☐ Neck
- ☐ Face
- ☐ Ears
- ☐ Eyes
- ☐ Nose
- ☐ Hair
- ☐ Mouth
- ☐ Jaw
- ☐ Teeth
- ☐ Tongue

Upper Body
- ☐ Shoulders
- ☐ Back
- ☐ Upper Back
- ☐ Lower Back
- ☐ Arms
- ☐ Elbows
- ☐ Hands
- ☐ Wrists
- ☐ Fingers
- ☐ Chest
- ☐ Sternum
- ☐ Torso

Lower Body
- ☐ Hips
- ☐ Bottom
- ☐ Legs
- ☐ Thighs
- ☐ Knees
- ☐ Calves
- ☐ Ankles
- ☐ Feet
- ☐ Toes

Sensory Systems
- ☐ Taste
- ☐ Smell
- ☐ Hearing
- ☐ Sight
- ☐ Throat

Other
- ☐ Mental
- ☐ _____
- ☐ _____
- ☐ _____
- ☐ _____
- ☐ _____
- ☐ _____

Describe the pain in your own words: _____

_____

_____

_____

_____

_____

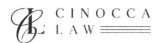

Date: _____   Day: _____

Severity of Pain

Morning: _____

Afternoon: _____

Evening: _____

Middle of Night: _____

Type of Pain   ☐ Throbbing   ☐ Aching   ☐ Stabbing   ☐ _____

Appetite: _____

Sleep: _____

Emotional Well Being

Mood Rating 1-10: _____

Emotional Issues: _____

_____

Nightmares: _____

Fears, Worries, Concerns: _____

_____

Observations

Changes in Symptoms: _____

Side Effects from Medications: _____

Improvements: _____

Deteriorations in Conditions: _____

Medications Taken When & Amount: _____

Limitations on Range of Motion: _____

Impairment of Daily Activities: _____

Help Needed: _____

_____

Help Received: _____

_____

NAME: _____

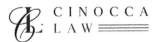 CINOCCA LAW

Date: _____   Day: _____

Appointments

Drs.: _____

Clinics: _____

Labs: _____

Therapy: _____

Pharmacy: _____

Visits: _____

Treatments: _____

Date: _____   Name: _____

Specialty: _____   Purpose: _____

Outcome: _____

_____

Conversations: _____

_____

Dr. Instructions: _____

_____

Date: _____   Name: _____

Specialty: _____   Purpose: _____

Outcome: _____

_____

Conversations: _____

_____

Dr. Instructions: _____

_____

Medication Name:	Strength/Dose:	When?
_____	_____	_____
_____	_____	_____
_____	_____	_____

NAME: _____

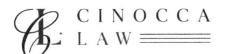
NAME: _____

DATE: _____   **DAYS POST INJURY:** _____

Body Areas Affected & How

Check any & all body parts affected by the accident:

Head and Neck

- ☐ Head
- ☐ Neck
- ☐ Face
- ☐ Ears
- ☐ Eyes
- ☐ Nose
- ☐ Hair
- ☐ Mouth
- ☐ Jaw
- ☐ Teeth
- ☐ Tongue

Upper Body

- ☐ Shoulders
- ☐ Back
- ☐ Upper Back
- ☐ Lower Back
- ☐ Arms
- ☐ Elbows
- ☐ Hands
- ☐ Wrists
- ☐ Fingers
- ☐ Chest
- ☐ Sternum
- ☐ Torso

Lower Body

- ☐ Hips
- ☐ Bottom
- ☐ Legs
- ☐ Thighs
- ☐ Knees
- ☐ Calves
- ☐ Ankles
- ☐ Feet
- ☐ Toes

Sensory Systems

- ☐ Taste
- ☐ Smell
- ☐ Hearing
- ☐ Sight
- ☐ Throat

Other

- ☐ Mental
- ☐ _____
- ☐ _____
- ☐ _____
- ☐ _____
- ☐ _____
- ☐ _____

Describe the pain in your own words: _____

_____

_____

_____

_____

_____

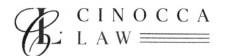

CINOCCA
LAW

NAME: _____

DATE: _____   **DAYS POST INJURY:** _____

Body Areas Affected & How

Check any & all body parts affected by the accident:

Head and Neck
- ☐ Head
- ☐ Neck
- ☐ Face
- ☐ Ears
- ☐ Eyes
- ☐ Nose
- ☐ Hair
- ☐ Mouth
- ☐ Jaw
- ☐ Teeth
- ☐ Tongue

Upper Body
- ☐ Shoulders
- ☐ Back
- ☐ Upper Back
- ☐ Lower Back
- ☐ Arms
- ☐ Elbows
- ☐ Hands
- ☐ Wrists
- ☐ Fingers
- ☐ Chest
- ☐ Sternum
- ☐ Torso

Lower Body
- ☐ Hips
- ☐ Bottom
- ☐ Legs
- ☐ Thighs
- ☐ Knees
- ☐ Calves
- ☐ Ankles
- ☐ Feet
- ☐ Toes

Sensory Systems
- ☐ Taste
- ☐ Smell
- ☐ Hearing
- ☐ Sight
- ☐ Throat

Other
- ☐ Mental
- ☐ _____
- ☐ _____
- ☐ _____
- ☐ _____
- ☐ _____
- ☐ _____

Describe the pain in your own words: _____

_____

_____

_____

_____

_____

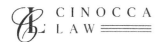

Date: _____   Day: _____

Severity of Pain

Morning: _____

Afternoon: _____

Evening: _____

Middle of Night: _____

Type of Pain   ☐ Throbbing   ☐ Aching   ☐ Stabbing   ☐ _____

Appetite: _____

Sleep: _____

Emotional Well Being

Mood Rating 1-10: _____

Emotional Issues: _____

_____

Nightmares: _____

Fears, Worries, Concerns: _____

_____

Observations

Changes in Symptoms: _____

Side Effects from Medications: _____

Improvements: _____

Deteriorations in Conditions: _____

Medications Taken When & Amount: _____

Limitations on Range of Motion: _____

Impairment of Daily Activities: _____

Help Needed: _____

_____

Help Received: _____

_____

NAME: _____

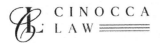

Date: _____ Day: _____

Appointments

Drs.: _____

Clinics: _____

Labs: _____

Therapy: _____

Pharmacy: _____

Visits: _____

Treatments: _____

Date: _____ Name: _____

Specialty: _____ Purpose: _____

Outcome: _____

_____

Conversations: _____

_____

Dr. Instructions: _____

_____

Date: _____ Name: _____

Specialty: _____ Purpose: _____

Outcome: _____

_____

Conversations: _____

_____

Dr. Instructions: _____

_____

Medication Name:	Strength/Dose:	When?
_____	_____	_____
_____	_____	_____
_____	_____	_____

NAME: _____

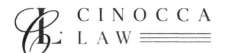

CINOCCA LAW

NAME: _____

DATE: _____ DAYS POST INJURY: _____

Body Areas Affected & How

Check any & all body parts affected by the accident:

Head and Neck

☐ Head
☐ Neck
☐ Face
☐ Ears
☐ Eyes
☐ Nose
☐ Hair
☐ Mouth
☐ Jaw
☐ Teeth
☐ Tongue

Upper Body

☐ Shoulders
☐ Back
☐ Upper Back
☐ Lower Back
☐ Arms
☐ Elbows
☐ Hands
☐ Wrists
☐ Fingers
☐ Chest
☐ Sternum
☐ Torso

Lower Body

☐ Hips
☐ Bottom
☐ Legs
☐ Thighs
☐ Knees
☐ Calves
☐ Ankles
☐ Feet
☐ Toes

Sensory Systems

☐ Taste
☐ Smell
☐ Hearing
☐ Sight
☐ Throat

Other

☐ Mental
☐ _____
☐ _____
☐ _____
☐ _____
☐ _____
☐ _____

Describe the pain in your own words: _____

_____

_____

_____

_____

_____

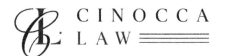
CINOCCA LAW

NAME: _____

DATE: _____   **DAYS POST INJURY:** _____

Body Areas Affected & How

Check any & all body parts affected by the accident:

Head and Neck
- ☐ Head
- ☐ Neck
- ☐ Face
- ☐ Ears
- ☐ Eyes
- ☐ Nose
- ☐ Hair
- ☐ Mouth
- ☐ Jaw
- ☐ Teeth
- ☐ Tongue

Upper Body
- ☐ Shoulders
- ☐ Back
- ☐ Upper Back
- ☐ Lower Back
- ☐ Arms
- ☐ Elbows
- ☐ Hands
- ☐ Wrists
- ☐ Fingers
- ☐ Chest
- ☐ Sternum
- ☐ Torso

Lower Body
- ☐ Hips
- ☐ Bottom
- ☐ Legs
- ☐ Thighs
- ☐ Knees
- ☐ Calves
- ☐ Ankles
- ☐ Feet
- ☐ Toes

Sensory Systems
- ☐ Taste
- ☐ Smell
- ☐ Hearing
- ☐ Sight
- ☐ Throat

Other
- ☐ Mental
- ☐ _____
- ☐ _____
- ☐ _____
- ☐ _____
- ☐ _____
- ☐ _____

Describe the pain in your own words: _____

_____

_____

_____

_____

_____

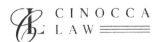

Date: _____ Day: _____

Severity of Pain

Morning: _____

Afternoon: _____

Evening: _____

Middle of Night: _____

Type of Pain ☐ Throbbing ☐ Aching ☐ Stabbing ☐ _____

Appetite: _____

Sleep: _____

Emotional Well Being

Mood Rating 1-10: _____

Emotional Issues: _____

_____

Nightmares: _____

Fears, Worries, Concerns: _____

_____

Observations

Changes in Symptoms: _____

Side Effects from Medications: _____

Improvements: _____

Deteriorations in Conditions: _____

Medications Taken When & Amount: _____

Limitations on Range of Motion: _____

Impairment of Daily Activities: _____

Help Needed: _____

_____

Help Received: _____

_____

NAME: _____

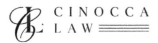

Date: _____ Day: _____

Appointments

Drs.: _____

Clinics: _____

Labs: _____

Therapy: _____

Pharmacy: _____

Visits: _____

Treatments: _____

Date: _____ Name: _____

Specialty: _____ Purpose: _____

Outcome: _____

_____

Conversations: _____

_____

Dr. Instructions: _____

_____

Date: _____ Name: _____

Specialty: _____ Purpose: _____

Outcome: _____

_____

Conversations: _____

_____

Dr. Instructions: _____

_____

Medication Name:	Strength/Dose:	When?
_____	_____	_____
_____	_____	_____
_____	_____	_____

NAME: _____

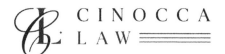

NAME: _____

DATE: _____   **DAYS POST INJURY:** _____

Body Areas Affected & How

Check any & all body parts affected by the accident:

Head and Neck

- ☐ Head
- ☐ Neck
- ☐ Face
- ☐ Ears
- ☐ Eyes
- ☐ Nose
- ☐ Hair
- ☐ Mouth
- ☐ Jaw
- ☐ Teeth
- ☐ Tongue

Upper Body

- ☐ Shoulders
- ☐ Back
- ☐ Upper Back
- ☐ Lower Back
- ☐ Arms
- ☐ Elbows
- ☐ Hands
- ☐ Wrists
- ☐ Fingers
- ☐ Chest
- ☐ Sternum
- ☐ Torso

Lower Body

- ☐ Hips
- ☐ Bottom
- ☐ Legs
- ☐ Thighs
- ☐ Knees
- ☐ Calves
- ☐ Ankles
- ☐ Feet
- ☐ Toes

Sensory Systems

- ☐ Taste
- ☐ Smell
- ☐ Hearing
- ☐ Sight
- ☐ Throat

Other

- ☐ Mental
- ☐ _____
- ☐ _____
- ☐ _____
- ☐ _____
- ☐ _____
- ☐ _____

Describe the pain in your own words: _____

_____

_____

_____

_____

_____

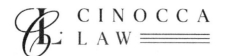

NAME: _____

DATE: _____   **DAYS POST INJURY:** _____

Body Areas Affected & How

Check any & all body parts affected by the accident:

Head and Neck
- ☐ Head
- ☐ Neck
- ☐ Face
- ☐ Ears
- ☐ Eyes
- ☐ Nose
- ☐ Hair
- ☐ Mouth
- ☐ Jaw
- ☐ Teeth
- ☐ Tongue

Upper Body
- ☐ Shoulders
- ☐ Back
- ☐ Upper Back
- ☐ Lower Back
- ☐ Arms
- ☐ Elbows
- ☐ Hands
- ☐ Wrists
- ☐ Fingers
- ☐ Chest
- ☐ Sternum
- ☐ Torso

Lower Body
- ☐ Hips
- ☐ Bottom
- ☐ Legs
- ☐ Thighs
- ☐ Knees
- ☐ Calves
- ☐ Ankles
- ☐ Feet
- ☐ Toes

Sensory Systems
- ☐ Taste
- ☐ Smell
- ☐ Hearing
- ☐ Sight
- ☐ Throat

Other
- ☐ Mental
- ☐ _____
- ☐ _____
- ☐ _____
- ☐ _____
- ☐ _____
- ☐ _____

Describe the pain in your own words: _____

_____

_____

_____

_____

_____

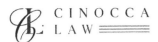

Date: _____ Day: _____

Severity of Pain

Morning: _____

Afternoon: _____

Evening: _____

Middle of Night: _____

Type of Pain ☐ Throbbing ☐ Aching ☐ Stabbing ☐ _____

Appetite: _____

Sleep: _____

Emotional Well Being

Mood Rating 1-10: _____

Emotional Issues: _____

_____

Nightmares: _____

Fears, Worries, Concerns: _____

_____

Observations

Changes in Symptoms: _____

Side Effects from Medications: _____

Improvements: _____

Deteriorations in Conditions: _____

Medications Taken When & Amount: _____

Limitations on Range of Motion: _____

Impairment of Daily Activities: _____

Help Needed: _____

_____

Help Received: _____

_____

NAME: _____

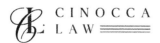

Date: _____ Day: _____

Appointments

Drs.: _____

Clinics: _____

Labs: _____

Therapy: _____

Pharmacy: _____

Visits: _____

Treatments: _____

Date: _____ Name: _____

Specialty: _____ Purpose: _____

Outcome: _____

_____

Conversations: _____

_____

Dr. Instructions: _____

_____

Date: _____ Name: _____

Specialty: _____ Purpose: _____

Outcome: _____

_____

Conversations: _____

_____

Dr. Instructions: _____

_____

Medication Name:	Strength/Dose:	When?
_____	_____	_____
_____	_____	_____
_____	_____	_____

NAME: _____

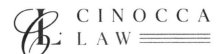

NAME: _____

DATE: _____   **DAYS POST INJURY:** _____

Body Areas Affected & How

Check any & all body parts affected by the accident:

Head and Neck

☐ Head
☐ Neck
☐ Face
☐ Ears
☐ Eyes
☐ Nose
☐ Hair
☐ Mouth
☐ Jaw
☐ Teeth
☐ Tongue

Upper Body

☐ Shoulders
☐ Back
☐ Upper Back
☐ Lower Back
☐ Arms
☐ Elbows
☐ Hands
☐ Wrists
☐ Fingers
☐ Chest
☐ Sternum
☐ Torso

Lower Body

☐ Hips
☐ Bottom
☐ Legs
☐ Thighs
☐ Knees
☐ Calves
☐ Ankles
☐ Feet
☐ Toes

Sensory Systems

☐ Taste
☐ Smell
☐ Hearing
☐ Sight
☐ Throat

Other

☐ Mental
☐ _____
☐ _____
☐ _____
☐ _____
☐ _____

Describe the pain in your own words: _____

_____

_____

_____

_____

_____

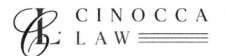

NAME: _____

DATE: _____   **DAYS POST INJURY:** _____

Body Areas Affected & How

Check any & all body parts affected by the accident:

Head and Neck
- ☐ Head
- ☐ Neck
- ☐ Face
- ☐ Ears
- ☐ Eyes
- ☐ Nose
- ☐ Hair
- ☐ Mouth
- ☐ Jaw
- ☐ Teeth
- ☐ Tongue

Upper Body
- ☐ Shoulders
- ☐ Back
- ☐ Upper Back
- ☐ Lower Back
- ☐ Arms
- ☐ Elbows
- ☐ Hands
- ☐ Wrists
- ☐ Fingers
- ☐ Chest
- ☐ Sternum
- ☐ Torso

Lower Body
- ☐ Hips
- ☐ Bottom
- ☐ Legs
- ☐ Thighs
- ☐ Knees
- ☐ Calves
- ☐ Ankles
- ☐ Feet
- ☐ Toes

Sensory Systems
- ☐ Taste
- ☐ Smell
- ☐ Hearing
- ☐ Sight
- ☐ Throat

Other
- ☐ Mental
- ☐ _____
- ☐ _____
- ☐ _____
- ☐ _____
- ☐ _____
- ☐ _____

Describe the pain in your own words: _____

_____

_____

_____

_____

_____

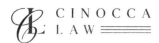

Date: _____ Day: _____

Severity of Pain

Morning: _____

Afternoon: _____

Evening: _____

Middle of Night: _____

Type of Pain   ☐ Throbbing   ☐ Aching   ☐ Stabbing   ☐ _____

Appetite: _____

Sleep: _____

Emotional Well Being

Mood Rating 1-10: _____

Emotional Issues: _____

_____

Nightmares: _____

Fears, Worries, Concerns: _____

_____

Observations

Changes in Symptoms: _____

Side Effects from Medications: _____

Improvements: _____

Deteriorations in Conditions: _____

Medications Taken When & Amount: _____

Limitations on Range of Motion: _____

Impairment of Daily Activities: _____

Help Needed: _____

_____

Help Received: _____

_____

NAME: _____

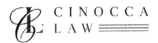

Appointments

Drs.: _____

Clinics: _____

Labs: _____

Therapy: _____

Pharmacy: _____

Visits: _____

Treatments: _____

Date: _____ Name: _____

Specialty: _____ Purpose: _____

Outcome: _____

_____

Conversations: _____

_____

Dr. Instructions: _____

_____

Date: _____ Name: _____

Specialty: _____ Purpose: _____

Outcome: _____

_____

Conversations: _____

_____

Dr. Instructions: _____

_____

Medication Name:	Strength/Dose:	When?
_____	_____	_____
_____	_____	_____
_____	_____	_____

NAME: _____

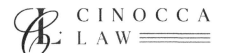

Personal and Confidential Communication Subject to Attorney Client and Work Product Privilege

NAME: _____

DATE: _____ **DAYS POST INJURY:** _____

Body Areas Affected & How

Check any & all body parts affected by the accident:

Head and Neck

- ☐ Head
- ☐ Neck
- ☐ Face
- ☐ Ears
- ☐ Eyes
- ☐ Nose
- ☐ Hair
- ☐ Mouth
- ☐ Jaw
- ☐ Teeth
- ☐ Tongue

Upper Body

- ☐ Shoulders
- ☐ Back
- ☐ Upper Back
- ☐ Lower Back
- ☐ Arms
- ☐ Elbows
- ☐ Hands
- ☐ Wrists
- ☐ Fingers
- ☐ Chest
- ☐ Sternum
- ☐ Torso

Lower Body

- ☐ Hips
- ☐ Bottom
- ☐ Legs
- ☐ Thighs
- ☐ Knees
- ☐ Calves
- ☐ Ankles
- ☐ Feet
- ☐ Toes

Sensory Systems

- ☐ Taste
- ☐ Smell
- ☐ Hearing
- ☐ Sight
- ☐ Throat

Other

- ☐ Mental
- ☐ _____
- ☐ _____
- ☐ _____
- ☐ _____
- ☐ _____
- ☐ _____

Describe the pain in your own words: _____

_____

_____

_____

_____

_____

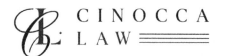

CINOCCA LAW

Personal and Confidential Communication Subject to Attorney Client and Work Product Privilege

NAME: _____

DATE: _____ **DAYS POST INJURY:** _____

Body Areas Affected & How

Check any & all body parts affected by the accident:

Head and Neck
- ☐ Head
- ☐ Neck
- ☐ Face
- ☐ Ears
- ☐ Eyes
- ☐ Nose
- ☐ Hair
- ☐ Mouth
- ☐ Jaw
- ☐ Teeth
- ☐ Tongue

Upper Body
- ☐ Shoulders
- ☐ Back
- ☐ Upper Back
- ☐ Lower Back
- ☐ Arms
- ☐ Elbows
- ☐ Hands
- ☐ Wrists
- ☐ Fingers
- ☐ Chest
- ☐ Sternum
- ☐ Torso

Lower Body
- ☐ Hips
- ☐ Bottom
- ☐ Legs
- ☐ Thighs
- ☐ Knees
- ☐ Calves
- ☐ Ankles
- ☐ Feet
- ☐ Toes

Sensory Systems
- ☐ Taste
- ☐ Smell
- ☐ Hearing
- ☐ Sight
- ☐ Throat

Other
- ☐ Mental
- ☐ _____
- ☐ _____
- ☐ _____
- ☐ _____
- ☐ _____
- ☐ _____

Describe the pain in your own words: _____

_____

_____

_____

_____

_____

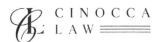

Date: _____   Day: _____

Severity of Pain

Morning: _____

Afternoon: _____

Evening: _____

Middle of Night: _____

Type of Pain   ☐ Throbbing   ☐ Aching   ☐ Stabbing   ☐ _____

Appetite: _____

Sleep: _____

Emotional Well Being

Mood Rating 1-10: _____

Emotional Issues: _____

_____

Nightmares: _____

Fears, Worries, Concerns: _____

_____

Observations

Changes in Symptoms: _____

Side Effects from Medications: _____

Improvements: _____

Deteriorations in Conditions: _____

Medications Taken When & Amount: _____

Limitations on Range of Motion: _____

Impairment of Daily Activities: _____

Help Needed: _____

_____

Help Received: _____

_____

NAME: _____

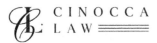

Appointments

Drs.: _____

Clinics: _____

Labs: _____

Therapy: _____

Pharmacy: _____

Visits: _____

Treatments: _____

Date: _____ Name: _____

Specialty: _____ Purpose: _____

Outcome: _____

_____

Conversations: _____

_____

Dr. Instructions: _____

_____

Date: _____ Name: _____

Specialty: _____ Purpose: _____

Outcome: _____

_____

Conversations: _____

_____

Dr. Instructions: _____

_____

Medication Name:	Strength/Dose:	When?
_____	_____	_____
_____	_____	_____
_____	_____	_____

NAME: _____

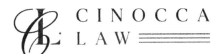

NAME: _____

DATE: _____   **DAYS POST INJURY:** _____

Body Areas Affected & How

Check any & all body parts affected by the accident:

Head and Neck

- ☐ Head
- ☐ Neck
- ☐ Face
- ☐ Ears
- ☐ Eyes
- ☐ Nose
- ☐ Hair
- ☐ Mouth
- ☐ Jaw
- ☐ Teeth
- ☐ Tongue

Upper Body

- ☐ Shoulders
- ☐ Back
- ☐ Upper Back
- ☐ Lower Back
- ☐ Arms
- ☐ Elbows
- ☐ Hands
- ☐ Wrists
- ☐ Fingers
- ☐ Chest
- ☐ Sternum
- ☐ Torso

Lower Body

- ☐ Hips
- ☐ Bottom
- ☐ Legs
- ☐ Thighs
- ☐ Knees
- ☐ Calves
- ☐ Ankles
- ☐ Feet
- ☐ Toes

Sensory Systems

- ☐ Taste
- ☐ Smell
- ☐ Hearing
- ☐ Sight
- ☐ Throat

Other

- ☐ Mental
- ☐ _____
- ☐ _____
- ☐ _____
- ☐ _____
- ☐ _____
- ☐ _____

Describe the pain in your own words: _____

_____

_____

_____

_____

_____

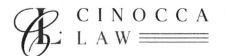

CINOCCA
LAW

Personal and Confidential Communication Subject to
Attorney Client and Work Product Privilege

NAME: _____

DATE: _____   **DAYS POST INJURY:** _____

Body Areas Affected & How

Check any & all body parts affected by the accident:

Head and Neck
- ☐ Head
- ☐ Neck
- ☐ Face
- ☐ Ears
- ☐ Eyes
- ☐ Nose
- ☐ Hair
- ☐ Mouth
- ☐ Jaw
- ☐ Teeth
- ☐ Tongue

Upper Body
- ☐ Shoulders
- ☐ Back
- ☐ Upper Back
- ☐ Lower Back
- ☐ Arms
- ☐ Elbows
- ☐ Hands
- ☐ Wrists
- ☐ Fingers
- ☐ Chest
- ☐ Sternum
- ☐ Torso

Lower Body
- ☐ Hips
- ☐ Bottom
- ☐ Legs
- ☐ Thighs
- ☐ Knees
- ☐ Calves
- ☐ Ankles
- ☐ Feet
- ☐ Toes

Sensory Systems
- ☐ Taste
- ☐ Smell
- ☐ Hearing
- ☐ Sight
- ☐ Throat

Other
- ☐ Mental
- ☐ _____
- ☐ _____
- ☐ _____
- ☐ _____
- ☐ _____
- ☐ _____

Describe the pain in your own words: _____

_____

_____

_____

_____

_____

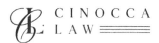

Date: _____   Day: _____

Severity of Pain

Morning: _____

Afternoon: _____

Evening: _____

Middle of Night: _____

Type of Pain   ☐ Throbbing   ☐ Aching   ☐ Stabbing   ☐ _____

Appetite: _____

Sleep: _____

Emotional Well Being

Mood Rating 1-10: _____

Emotional Issues: _____

_____

Nightmares: _____

Fears, Worries, Concerns: _____

_____

Observations

Changes in Symptoms: _____

Side Effects from Medications: _____

Improvements: _____

Deteriorations in Conditions: _____

Medications Taken When & Amount: _____

Limitations on Range of Motion: _____

Impairment of Daily Activities: _____

Help Needed: _____

_____

Help Received: _____

_____

NAME: _____

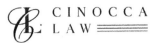

Date: _____ Day: _____

Appointments

Drs.: _____

Clinics: _____

Labs: _____

Therapy: _____

Pharmacy: _____

Visits: _____

Treatments: _____

Date: _____ Name: _____

Specialty: _____ Purpose: _____

Outcome: _____

_____

Conversations: _____

_____

Dr. Instructions: _____

_____

Date: _____ Name: _____

Specialty: _____ Purpose: _____

Outcome: _____

_____

Conversations: _____

_____

Dr. Instructions: _____

_____

Medication Name:	Strength/Dose:	When?
_____	_____	_____
_____	_____	_____
_____	_____	_____

NAME: _____

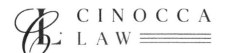

Personal and Confidential Communication Subject to
Attorney Client and Work Product Privilege

NAME: _____

DATE: _____   **DAYS POST INJURY:** _____

Body Areas Affected & How

Check any & all body parts affected by the accident:

Head and Neck

- ☐ Head
- ☐ Neck
- ☐ Face
- ☐ Ears
- ☐ Eyes
- ☐ Nose
- ☐ Hair
- ☐ Mouth
- ☐ Jaw
- ☐ Teeth
- ☐ Tongue

Upper Body

- ☐ Shoulders
- ☐ Back
- ☐ Upper Back
- ☐ Lower Back
- ☐ Arms
- ☐ Elbows
- ☐ Hands
- ☐ Wrists
- ☐ Fingers
- ☐ Chest
- ☐ Sternum
- ☐ Torso

Lower Body

- ☐ Hips
- ☐ Bottom
- ☐ Legs
- ☐ Thighs
- ☐ Knees
- ☐ Calves
- ☐ Ankles
- ☐ Feet
- ☐ Toes

Sensory Systems

- ☐ Taste
- ☐ Smell
- ☐ Hearing
- ☐ Sight
- ☐ Throat

Other

- ☐ Mental
- ☐ _____
- ☐ _____
- ☐ _____
- ☐ _____
- ☐ _____
- ☐ _____

Describe the pain in your own words: _____

_____

_____

_____

_____

_____

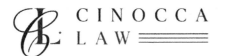
CINOCCA LAW

NAME: _____

DATE: _____ **DAYS POST INJURY:** _____

Body Areas Affected & How

Check any & all body parts affected by the accident:

Head and Neck
- ☐ Head
- ☐ Neck
- ☐ Face
- ☐ Ears
- ☐ Eyes
- ☐ Nose
- ☐ Hair
- ☐ Mouth
- ☐ Jaw
- ☐ Teeth
- ☐ Tongue

Upper Body
- ☐ Shoulders
- ☐ Back
- ☐ Upper Back
- ☐ Lower Back
- ☐ Arms
- ☐ Elbows
- ☐ Hands
- ☐ Wrists
- ☐ Fingers
- ☐ Chest
- ☐ Sternum
- ☐ Torso

Lower Body
- ☐ Hips
- ☐ Bottom
- ☐ Legs
- ☐ Thighs
- ☐ Knees
- ☐ Calves
- ☐ Ankles
- ☐ Feet
- ☐ Toes

Sensory Systems
- ☐ Taste
- ☐ Smell
- ☐ Hearing
- ☐ Sight
- ☐ Throat

Other
- ☐ Mental
- ☐ _____
- ☐ _____
- ☐ _____
- ☐ _____
- ☐ _____
- ☐ _____

Describe the pain in your own words: _____

_____

_____

_____

_____

_____

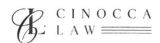

Date: _____ Day: _____

Severity of Pain

Morning: _____

Afternoon: _____

Evening: _____

Middle of Night: _____

Type of Pain   ☐ Throbbing   ☐ Aching   ☐ Stabbing   ☐ _____

Appetite: _____

Sleep: _____

Emotional Well Being

Mood Rating 1-10: _____

Emotional Issues: _____

_____

Nightmares: _____

Fears, Worries, Concerns: _____

_____

Observations

Changes in Symptoms: _____

Side Effects from Medications: _____

Improvements: _____

Deteriorations in Conditions: _____

Medications Taken When & Amount: _____

Limitations on Range of Motion: _____

Impairment of Daily Activities: _____

Help Needed: _____

_____

Help Received: _____

_____

NAME: _____

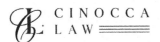

Date: _____   Day: _____

Appointments

Drs.: _____

Clinics: _____

Labs: _____

Therapy: _____

Pharmacy: _____

Visits: _____

Treatments: _____

Date: _____   Name: _____

Specialty: _____   Purpose: _____

Outcome: _____

_____

Conversations: _____

_____

Dr. Instructions: _____

_____

Date: _____   Name: _____

Specialty: _____   Purpose: _____

Outcome: _____

_____

Conversations: _____

_____

Dr. Instructions: _____

_____

Medication Name:	Strength/Dose:	When?
_____	_____	_____
_____	_____	_____
_____	_____	_____

NAME: _____

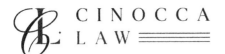

CINOCCA
LAW

Personal and Confidential Communication Subject to Attorney Client and Work Product Privilege

NAME: _____

DATE: _____ **DAYS POST INJURY:** _____

Body Areas Affected & How

Check any & all body parts affected by the accident:

Head and Neck

- ☐ Head
- ☐ Neck
- ☐ Face
- ☐ Ears
- ☐ Eyes
- ☐ Nose
- ☐ Hair
- ☐ Mouth
- ☐ Jaw
- ☐ Teeth
- ☐ Tongue

Upper Body

- ☐ Shoulders
- ☐ Back
- ☐ Upper Back
- ☐ Lower Back
- ☐ Arms
- ☐ Elbows
- ☐ Hands
- ☐ Wrists
- ☐ Fingers
- ☐ Chest
- ☐ Sternum
- ☐ Torso

Lower Body

- ☐ Hips
- ☐ Bottom
- ☐ Legs
- ☐ Thighs
- ☐ Knees
- ☐ Calves
- ☐ Ankles
- ☐ Feet
- ☐ Toes

Sensory Systems

- ☐ Taste
- ☐ Smell
- ☐ Hearing
- ☐ Sight
- ☐ Throat

Other

- ☐ Mental
- ☐ _____
- ☐ _____
- ☐ _____
- ☐ _____
- ☐ _____
- ☐ _____

Describe the pain in your own words: _____

_____

_____

_____

_____

_____

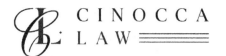

NAME: _____

DATE: _____   **DAYS POST INJURY:** _____

Body Areas Affected & How

Check any & all body parts affected by the accident:

Head and Neck
- ☐ Head
- ☐ Neck
- ☐ Face
- ☐ Ears
- ☐ Eyes
- ☐ Nose
- ☐ Hair
- ☐ Mouth
- ☐ Jaw
- ☐ Teeth
- ☐ Tongue

Upper Body
- ☐ Shoulders
- ☐ Back
- ☐ Upper Back
- ☐ Lower Back
- ☐ Arms
- ☐ Elbows
- ☐ Hands
- ☐ Wrists
- ☐ Fingers
- ☐ Chest
- ☐ Sternum
- ☐ Torso

Lower Body
- ☐ Hips
- ☐ Bottom
- ☐ Legs
- ☐ Thighs
- ☐ Knees
- ☐ Calves
- ☐ Ankles
- ☐ Feet
- ☐ Toes

Sensory Systems
- ☐ Taste
- ☐ Smell
- ☐ Hearing
- ☐ Sight
- ☐ Throat

Other
- ☐ Mental
- ☐ _____
- ☐ _____
- ☐ _____
- ☐ _____
- ☐ _____
- ☐ _____

Describe the pain in your own words: _____

_____

_____

_____

_____

_____

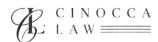

Date: _____ Day: _____

Severity of Pain

Morning: _____

Afternoon: _____

Evening: _____

Middle of Night: _____

Type of Pain ☐ Throbbing ☐ Aching ☐ Stabbing ☐ _____

Appetite: _____

Sleep: _____

Emotional Well Being

Mood Rating 1-10: _____

Emotional Issues: _____

_____

Nightmares: _____

Fears, Worries, Concerns: _____

_____

Observations

Changes in Symptoms: _____

Side Effects from Medications: _____

Improvements: _____

Deteriorations in Conditions: _____

Medications Taken When & Amount: _____

Limitations on Range of Motion: _____

Impairment of Daily Activities: _____

Help Needed: _____

_____

Help Received: _____

_____

NAME: _____

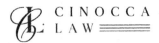

Date: _____ Day: _____

Appointments

Drs.: _____

Clinics: _____

Labs: _____

Therapy: _____

Pharmacy: _____

Visits: _____

Treatments: _____

Date: _____ Name: _____

Specialty: _____ Purpose: _____

Outcome: _____

_____

Conversations: _____

_____

Dr. Instructions: _____

_____

Date: _____ Name: _____

Specialty: _____ Purpose: _____

Outcome: _____

_____

Conversations: _____

_____

Dr. Instructions: _____

_____

Medication Name:	Strength/Dose:	When?
_____	_____	_____
_____	_____	_____
_____	_____	_____

NAME: _____

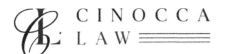

NAME: _____

DATE: _____   **DAYS POST INJURY:** _____

Body Areas Affected & How

Check any & all body parts affected by the accident:

Head and Neck

- ☐ Head
- ☐ Neck
- ☐ Face
- ☐ Ears
- ☐ Eyes
- ☐ Nose
- ☐ Hair
- ☐ Mouth
- ☐ Jaw
- ☐ Teeth
- ☐ Tongue

Upper Body

- ☐ Shoulders
- ☐ Back
- ☐ Upper Back
- ☐ Lower Back
- ☐ Arms
- ☐ Elbows
- ☐ Hands
- ☐ Wrists
- ☐ Fingers
- ☐ Chest
- ☐ Sternum
- ☐ Torso

Lower Body

- ☐ Hips
- ☐ Bottom
- ☐ Legs
- ☐ Thighs
- ☐ Knees
- ☐ Calves
- ☐ Ankles
- ☐ Feet
- ☐ Toes

Sensory Systems

- ☐ Taste
- ☐ Smell
- ☐ Hearing
- ☐ Sight
- ☐ Throat

Other

- ☐ Mental
- ☐ _____
- ☐ _____
- ☐ _____
- ☐ _____
- ☐ _____
- ☐ _____

Describe the pain in your own words: _____

_____

_____

_____

_____

_____

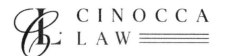

NAME: _____

DATE: _____ **DAYS POST INJURY:** _____

Body Areas Affected & How

Check any & all body parts affected by the accident:

Head and Neck
- ☐ Head
- ☐ Neck
- ☐ Face
- ☐ Ears
- ☐ Eyes
- ☐ Nose
- ☐ Hair
- ☐ Mouth
- ☐ Jaw
- ☐ Teeth
- ☐ Tongue

Upper Body
- ☐ Shoulders
- ☐ Back
- ☐ Upper Back
- ☐ Lower Back
- ☐ Arms
- ☐ Elbows
- ☐ Hands
- ☐ Wrists
- ☐ Fingers
- ☐ Chest
- ☐ Sternum
- ☐ Torso

Lower Body
- ☐ Hips
- ☐ Bottom
- ☐ Legs
- ☐ Thighs
- ☐ Knees
- ☐ Calves
- ☐ Ankles
- ☐ Feet
- ☐ Toes

Sensory Systems
- ☐ Taste
- ☐ Smell
- ☐ Hearing
- ☐ Sight
- ☐ Throat

Other
- ☐ Mental
- ☐ _____
- ☐ _____
- ☐ _____
- ☐ _____
- ☐ _____
- ☐ _____

Describe the pain in your own words: _____

_____

_____

_____

_____

_____

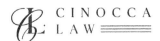

Date: _____ Day: _____

Severity of Pain

Morning: _____

Afternoon: _____

Evening: _____

Middle of Night: _____

Type of Pain ☐ Throbbing ☐ Aching ☐ Stabbing ☐ _____

Appetite: _____

Sleep: _____

Emotional Well Being

Mood Rating 1-10: _____

Emotional Issues: _____

_____

Nightmares: _____

Fears, Worries, Concerns: _____

_____

Observations

Changes in Symptoms: _____

Side Effects from Medications: _____

Improvements: _____

Deteriorations in Conditions: _____

Medications Taken When & Amount: _____

Limitations on Range of Motion: _____

Impairment of Daily Activities: _____

Help Needed: _____

_____

Help Received: _____

_____

NAME: _____

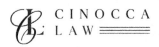

CINOCCA
LAW

Date: _____ Day: _____

Appointments

Drs.: _____

Clinics: _____

Labs: _____

Therapy: _____

Pharmacy: _____

Visits: _____

Treatments: _____

Date: _____ Name: _____

Specialty: _____ Purpose: _____

Outcome: _____

_____

Conversations: _____

_____

Dr. Instructions: _____

_____

Date: _____ Name: _____

Specialty: _____ Purpose: _____

Outcome: _____

_____

Conversations: _____

_____

Dr. Instructions: _____

_____

Medication Name:	Strength/Dose:	When?
_____	_____	_____
_____	_____	_____
_____	_____	_____

NAME: _____

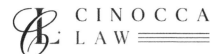

Personal and Confidential Communication Subject to Attorney Client and Work Product Privilege

NAME: _____

DATE: _____   **DAYS POST INJURY:** _____

Body Areas Affected & How

Check any & all body parts affected by the accident:

Head and Neck

- ☐ Head
- ☐ Neck
- ☐ Face
- ☐ Ears
- ☐ Eyes
- ☐ Nose
- ☐ Hair
- ☐ Mouth
- ☐ Jaw
- ☐ Teeth
- ☐ Tongue

Upper Body

- ☐ Shoulders
- ☐ Back
- ☐ Upper Back
- ☐ Lower Back
- ☐ Arms
- ☐ Elbows
- ☐ Hands
- ☐ Wrists
- ☐ Fingers
- ☐ Chest
- ☐ Sternum
- ☐ Torso

Lower Body

- ☐ Hips
- ☐ Bottom
- ☐ Legs
- ☐ Thighs
- ☐ Knees
- ☐ Calves
- ☐ Ankles
- ☐ Feet
- ☐ Toes

Sensory Systems

- ☐ Taste
- ☐ Smell
- ☐ Hearing
- ☐ Sight
- ☐ Throat

Other

- ☐ Mental
- ☐ _____
- ☐ _____
- ☐ _____
- ☐ _____
- ☐ _____
- ☐ _____

Describe the pain in your own words: _____

_____

_____

_____

_____

_____

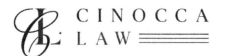
CINOCCA
LAW

NAME: _____

DATE: _____   **DAYS POST INJURY:** _____

Body Areas Affected & How

Check any & all body parts affected by the accident:

Head and Neck
- ☐ Head
- ☐ Neck
- ☐ Face
- ☐ Ears
- ☐ Eyes
- ☐ Nose
- ☐ Hair
- ☐ Mouth
- ☐ Jaw
- ☐ Teeth
- ☐ Tongue

Upper Body
- ☐ Shoulders
- ☐ Back
- ☐ Upper Back
- ☐ Lower Back
- ☐ Arms
- ☐ Elbows
- ☐ Hands
- ☐ Wrists
- ☐ Fingers
- ☐ Chest
- ☐ Sternum
- ☐ Torso

Lower Body
- ☐ Hips
- ☐ Bottom
- ☐ Legs
- ☐ Thighs
- ☐ Knees
- ☐ Calves
- ☐ Ankles
- ☐ Feet
- ☐ Toes

Sensory Systems
- ☐ Taste
- ☐ Smell
- ☐ Hearing
- ☐ Sight
- ☐ Throat

Other
- ☐ Mental
- ☐ _____
- ☐ _____
- ☐ _____
- ☐ _____
- ☐ _____
- ☐ _____

Describe the pain in your own words: _____

_____

_____

_____

_____

_____

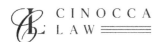

Date: _____ Day: _____

Severity of Pain

Morning: _____

Afternoon: _____

Evening: _____

Middle of Night: _____

Type of Pain ☐ Throbbing ☐ Aching ☐ Stabbing ☐ _____

Appetite: _____

Sleep: _____

Emotional Well Being

Mood Rating 1-10: _____

Emotional Issues: _____

_____

Nightmares: _____

Fears, Worries, Concerns: _____

_____

Observations

Changes in Symptoms: _____

Side Effects from Medications: _____

Improvements: _____

Deteriorations in Conditions: _____

Medications Taken When & Amount: _____

Limitations on Range of Motion: _____

Impairment of Daily Activities: _____

Help Needed: _____

_____

Help Received: _____

_____

NAME: _____

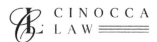

Date: _____   Day: _____

Appointments

Drs.:_____

Clinics: _____

Labs: _____

Therapy: _____

Pharmacy: _____

Visits: _____

Treatments:_____

Date: _____   Name: _____

Specialty: _____   Purpose: _____

Outcome: _____

_____

Conversations: _____

_____

Dr. Instructions: _____

_____

Date: _____   Name: _____

Specialty: _____   Purpose: _____

Outcome: _____

_____

Conversations: _____

_____

Dr. Instructions: _____

_____

Medication Name:	Strength/Dose:	When?
_____	_____	_____
_____	_____	_____
_____	_____	_____

NAME: _____

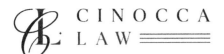
CINOCCA LAW

Personal and Confidential Communication Subject to Attorney Client and Work Product Privilege

NAME: _____

DATE: _____ **DAYS POST INJURY:** _____

Body Areas Affected & How

Check any & all body parts affected by the accident:

Head and Neck

- ☐ Head
- ☐ Neck
- ☐ Face
- ☐ Ears
- ☐ Eyes
- ☐ Nose
- ☐ Hair
- ☐ Mouth
- ☐ Jaw
- ☐ Teeth
- ☐ Tongue

Upper Body

- ☐ Shoulders
- ☐ Back
- ☐ Upper Back
- ☐ Lower Back
- ☐ Arms
- ☐ Elbows
- ☐ Hands
- ☐ Wrists
- ☐ Fingers
- ☐ Chest
- ☐ Sternum
- ☐ Torso

Lower Body

- ☐ Hips
- ☐ Bottom
- ☐ Legs
- ☐ Thighs
- ☐ Knees
- ☐ Calves
- ☐ Ankles
- ☐ Feet
- ☐ Toes

Sensory Systems

- ☐ Taste
- ☐ Smell
- ☐ Hearing
- ☐ Sight
- ☐ Throat

Other

- ☐ Mental
- ☐ _____
- ☐ _____
- ☐ _____
- ☐ _____
- ☐ _____
- ☐ _____

Describe the pain in your own words: _____

_____

_____

_____

_____

_____

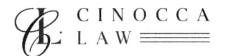

NAME: _____

DATE: _____   **DAYS POST INJURY:** _____

Body Areas Affected & How

Check any & all body parts affected by the accident:

Head and Neck

☐ Head
☐ Neck
☐ Face
☐ Ears
☐ Eyes
☐ Nose
☐ Hair
☐ Mouth
☐ Jaw
☐ Teeth
☐ Tongue

Upper Body

☐ Shoulders
☐ Back
☐ Upper Back
☐ Lower Back
☐ Arms
☐ Elbows
☐ Hands
☐ Wrists
☐ Fingers
☐ Chest
☐ Sternum
☐ Torso

Lower Body

☐ Hips
☐ Bottom
☐ Legs
☐ Thighs
☐ Knees
☐ Calves
☐ Ankles
☐ Feet
☐ Toes

Sensory Systems

☐ Taste
☐ Smell
☐ Hearing
☐ Sight
☐ Throat

Other

☐ Mental
☐ _____
☐ _____
☐ _____
☐ _____
☐ _____
☐ _____

Describe the pain in your own words: _____

_____

_____

_____

_____

_____

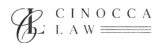

Date: _____ Day: _____

Severity of Pain

Morning: _____

Afternoon: _____

Evening: _____

Middle of Night: _____

Type of Pain ☐ Throbbing ☐ Aching ☐ Stabbing ☐ _____

Appetite: _____

Sleep: _____

Emotional Well Being

Mood Rating 1-10: _____

Emotional Issues: _____

_____

Nightmares: _____

Fears, Worries, Concerns: _____

_____

Observations

Changes in Symptoms: _____

Side Effects from Medications: _____

Improvements: _____

Deteriorations in Conditions: _____

Medications Taken When & Amount: _____

Limitations on Range of Motion: _____

Impairment of Daily Activities: _____

Help Needed: _____

_____

Help Received: _____

_____

NAME: _____

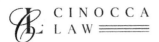

Date: _____ Day: _____

Appointments

Drs.: _____

Clinics: _____

Labs: _____

Therapy: _____

Pharmacy: _____

Visits: _____

Treatments: _____

Date: _____ Name: _____

Specialty: _____ Purpose: _____

Outcome: _____

_____

Conversations: _____

_____

Dr. Instructions: _____

_____

Date: _____ Name: _____

Specialty: _____ Purpose: _____

Outcome: _____

_____

Conversations: _____

_____

Dr. Instructions: _____

_____

Medication Name:	Strength/Dose:	When?
_____	_____	_____
_____	_____	_____
_____	_____	_____

NAME: _____

Made in the USA
Las Vegas, NV
08 May 2025